FRANKIE

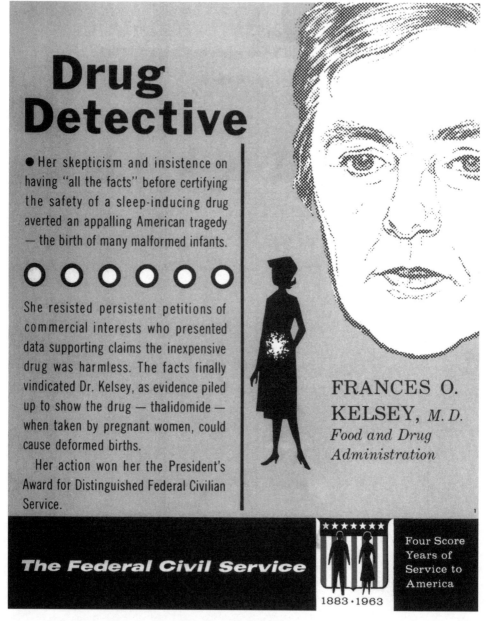

Frances Kelsey's steadfast refusal to approve thalidomide for the US market in the early 1960s attracted national attention, invoked in this recruitment poster for the US Civil Service. (US Food and Drug Administration)

FRANKIE

THE WOMAN WHO SAVED MILLIONS FROM THALIDOMIDE

JAMES ESSINGER & SANDRA KOUTZENKO

The History Press

To Briony Kapoor, in admiration. (JE)

To my grandmother Marie-Madeleine Sablery, whose own quiet
heroism taught me the true meaning of strength. (SK)

Originally published in the United States of America by Wellspring, 2019
First published in the UK 2019

The History Press
97 St George's Place, Cheltenham
Gloucestershire, GL50 3QB
www.thehistorypress.co.uk

British Library Cataloguing in Publication Data.
A catalogue record for this book is available from the British Library.

ISBN 978 0 7509 9191 9

Typesetting and origination by The History Press
Printed and bound in Great Britain by TJ International Ltd.

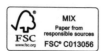

CONTENTS

'If thalidomide had been developed in this country,
I am convinced that it would easily have found wide distribution
before the terrible power to cause deformity had been apparent'.
Dr Helen Taussig in Scientific American, *August 1962*

'I was just absolutely shocked to hear that this drug company had
applied pressure on her [Frances Kelsey]. I mean it was outrageous,
pressurizing a medical officer of the FDA ... It was the first personal
awakening that really mattered as to what corporate conduct could be.
How bad it can be. How criminal it can be in some cases'.
Morton Mintz, interviewed on 27 April 2007,
by Professor Charles Lewis of The Investigative Reporting Workshop

'... thalidomide, the greatest drug tragedy ever known ...'
Sir Harold Evans in a letter to Dr Frances Kelsey (2015)

AUTHORS' NOTE

We mostly refer in this book to our heroine as 'Frankie'. We never had the pleasure and privilege of meeting her, which would in fact have been feasible, as she passed away comparatively recently, on 7 August 2015, aged 101. But we have had the privilege of being assisted in our research by people who knew Frances, in particular Dr John Swann, her former colleague at the United States Food and Drug Administration (FDA).

Even though we never met her, it seems excessively formal for us to refer to Frances here, in what is essentially an affectionate and admiring biography, as 'Frances', still less as 'Dr Kelsey', though we do use that name sometimes.

During her lifetime, she was known as Frankie by her parents, many of her schoolteachers, her husband, and many colleagues and friends. We hope that this book will give many more the opportunity to know this remarkable and brilliant woman, and so we've decided to refer to her informally as Frankie.

Please also note that all material contained in brackets is interpolations by the authors for clarity.

J.E. & S.K.

FOREWORD

by Sir Harold Evans

This biography has the excitement of mythical narrative and the relevance of the day's news feed. A young mother stands alone against Dark Forces ready to release disabling neurotoxins on our planet. She prevails by summoning the magical power of Truth – the eternal verity itself now under assault in post-truth societies that discount evidence in favor of fable and 'alternate' realities.

The heroine is Dr Frances Oldham Kelsey, the centenarian Frankie (1914–2015) of the authors' engaging title. She was in her forties working out of a bleak bare-floor office as a new medical officer at the Food and Drug Administration. Her first random assignment in 1960 was to agree to the distribution in America of a new 'wonder drug', now notorious as thalidomide. She found herself confronted by the imperial power of American business in the form of the pharmaceutical company, Richardson-Merrell. They expected her to rubber-stamp her approval of their submission. After all, thalidomide had already been patented in Germany and was being promoted by its makers as non-toxic, no side effects, completely non-poisonous, and safer than all other tranquilizers for relief in pregnancy from sleeplessness and morning sickness.

The Richardson-Merrell executives (all male) had 10 million pills ready for market. They represented a lottery of lies. Dependent on the day it was ingested, a single dose of thalidomide could kill babies in the womb, degrade their organs, or lop off limbs. The German inventors, Chemie Grünenthal, didn't know this, but they did ignore plenty of warning signs. They were new to pharmaceuticals, but other companies, including the liquor-makers Distillers in the UK, more or less took them on trust. Globally, thalidomide had eighty-nine different brand names: Contergan in Germany, Distaval in Britain, Kevadon in the US. Every one of them was poison.

The valiant thalidomiders of today with no arms, no legs, have made the best of lives devastated by the dangerous pill. They had faith in their doctors. Their doctors were betrayed by the incompetence and greed of the drugmakers. And then pretty well everywhere the devastated families were betrayed by the callous disregard of their governments.

This is the fate that would have been ordained for millions of Americans had Frankie not persisted. How did she prevail? She asked questions of Richardson-Merrell, good questions that got nowhere, as the authors track in exchanges from September 1960 to February 1961. For Frankie, a scientific truth must emerge from the most convincing evidence, and is always open to correction.

Frankie did not know what the precise catastrophic effects of thalidomide would be, but her scientific training was enough to alert her to the evidence that neurotoxins were likely to harm a fetus. Richardson-Merrell attacked her and the FDA for interfering with business. The questions infuriated Richardson-Merrell for a simple reason – they couldn't answer them. Nobody could, because none of the parties had done proper testing. One Kelsey memorandum is tellingly highlighted by the authors: 'We feel that we do not know enough about the metabolism and pharmacological effects of Contergan ...'

Her vigilance delayed the approval of the drug through November 1961, by which time hundreds of abnormal births had raised enough alarm for thalidomide to be withdrawn in Germany and Britain, though it was withdrawn more slowly in Canada and Spain.

At *The Sunday Times* in London, when we undertook an investigation of the deformed births, we were appalled that the drug, already approved by the National Health Service, was not even then subjected to a searching public inquiry of the kind that routinely attends disasters. The then UK health minister, Enoch Powell, sided with the delinquent drug company. So did his officials, Parliament, and Press. The chant they all took up was that thalidomide had been tested 'according to the standards of the time'. Nobody bothered to determine the reproductive standards of the world's best companies. The families were left to feel they had been punished by an unforeseeable act of God. Of course, it was said, they were free to seek compensation from the drug company. Good luck with that. When *The Sunday Times* set out to expose the miserable treatment of the families, the British government took us to court to suppress our findings.

We were inspired through many long years of prosecution and suppression by Frankie's shining example. It was a special, joyful moment for us to send her greetings on her hundredth birthday. 'Your heroism was twofold: one, in your insistence on the primacy of scientific evidence; two, in your courage in the face of incessant pressure from powerful interests. Happy 100th!'

The encounter between Frankie's reason and layers of assertion in law, business and government, took place somewhat more than half a century ago. Now there is a new neurotoxin in the air – one that affects the way we think. Great harm was done by propagation of the fraud that the MMR vaccine caused autism. Too many credulous people stopped vaccinating their children for measles because they were deluded into accepting the notion that the vaccine caused autism. People suffered because they believed fraudulent science. Let the story in this book heighten awareness of the symptoms of malaise in an appetite for fantasy, emotionally sustained in paranoid groups, disseminated in a flash, immune to reason and fact, susceptible to half-truths and lies.

Sir Harold Evans, as editor of The Sunday Times *(1967–1981), led the thalidomide investigation and the campaign that won compensation for victims. He is the author of* Good Times, Bad Times; My Paper Chase; *and* Do I Make Myself Clear? *and co-author of* Suffer the Children, *with Phil Knightley, Marjorie Wallace, and Elaine Potter.*

PROLOGUE

When we say someone looks like a poet, we don't mean they look like Shakespeare, nor like the Anglo-American poet T.S. Eliot, who spent many years of his career working in the city of London as a banker and was often photographed wearing a suit. Still less do we mean that they resemble Philip Larkin, the illustrious twentieth-century British poet, who as an adult was tall, skinny, balding and bespectacled.

No, when we say someone looks like a poet, we mean they remind us of Lord Byron or Percy Shelley. It's not clear why this cultural notion of the typical appearance of a poet has persisted from the Romantic Age of poetry of the late eighteenth and early nineteenth century, but it has.

We also tend, more generally, to have an archetype for what constitutes a person who makes a profoundly positive mark on the world. We usually adopt the attitude that such people are likely to be extroverted, comparatively brash – even loud – and intensely passionate about their work, and that people who are quieter and more introspective are less likely to be successful.

Our epoch places an emphasis on soundbites and easy-to-understand summaries of careers that have usually been far more complex, and far more troubled by setbacks, than the person's public image implies. Confusing achievement with the prominence of a person's image is a kind of cultural shorthand that can, too easily, falsify both history and living reality.

There is no clear cultural image today of what a hero or heroine should look like. This wasn't true of the Romans or the Greeks; they were quite sure that a hero (and their heroes were almost all men) would have tremendous musculature and abundant shining armor, and be blessed with tremendous physical skill in using deadly weaponry.

This book is about a woman called Frances Kelsey, a completely different kind of heroine. She is one of the most eminent women in the history of medicine, not only in the United States, but in the world, yet during the twentieth century she was not even given a mention in *Encyclopedia Britannica*. Nowadays she is.

It's reasonable to describe Frankie as a 'reluctant heroine', not because she didn't want to do the wonderful things she did, but because to her, what she did was simply part of her job. She didn't seek fame or prestige; still less did she set out to be regarded as a heroine. Yet all the same, she is one of the great heroines of history, and she did far more for humankind than any Greek or Roman hero ever did.

In modern culture, reluctant heroes are typically portrayed as ordinary people, thrust into extraordinary circumstances which require them to rise to a heroism they don't seek, but who rise to the challenge nonetheless and prove themselves abundantly worthy of the mantle fate has placed upon them.

Dr John Swann, a historian at the Food and Drug Administration (FDA) in Washington, D.C., who knew Dr Kelsey personally in her old age, comments:

Other people have made more of Frances's achievements than she did herself. She didn't dwell on what she'd done. As far as she was concerned, she'd been given a job and she applied herself to it with devotion and meticulous attention.

The world, not unreasonably, has taken a different view. Today, there are many tens of thousands of people living in the United States whose lives would have been irretrievably blighted had it not been for Frances.

As Matthew Kelly, the best-selling inspirational speaker and writer, comments:

> There are many ways to measure good; one of those ways, I believe, is to consider the suffering that would have occurred if that person had never existed or had never done their work.

This insightful remark offers a deep and ingenious way of defining heroism: a way which doesn't rely on the typical hero attributes (how actively one seeks to help others, or how much they are willing to sacrifice for the greater good), but instead focuses on the impact one has had upon the world. What Kelly is suggesting is that, alongside the world we inhabit, there is a darker world of disastrous events that never happened. Of course, there is also, within our world and our history, a darker world of disastrous events that *did* happen, and there are heroes and heroines who have acted to reduce the duration of these dark effects or to alleviate the suffering caused, but that's another matter.

In Dr Kelsey's case, the suffering that would have occurred if that person had never existed or had never done their work was due to a drug called thalidomide, sold in many countries around the world as a sedative and – tragically – as a highly effective cure for morning sickness in pregnant women. In fact, thalidomide was subsequently found to cause appalling physical injuries and deformities in babies while they were in the womb, damage that was in many cases so severe that the baby died before it even had a chance to be born.

When we think of the nature of Dr Kelsey's heroism, it is instructive and moving to consider a remarkable poem by John Milton, in which he reflects on the poor eyesight that started to afflict him from the age of around 36, in 1644. By early 1650 he had nearly lost his sight, mainly due, as he understood it, to his love of study and working by candlelight until late in the night. Unfortunately, Milton became completely blind during the winter of 1651–1652.

Milton probably dictated the sonnet to an assistant, as he most likely wrote it at a time when he had lost his sight completely.

> When I consider how my light is spent,
>
> Ere half my days in this dark world and wide,
>
> And that one talent which is death to hide
>
> Lodged with me useless, though my soul more bent
>
> To serve therewith my Maker, and present
>
> My true account, lest he returning chide;
>
> 'Doth God exact day-labor, light denied?'
>
> I fondly ask. But Patience to prevent
>
> That murmur, soon replies: 'God doth not need
>
> Either man's work or his own gifts; who best
>
> Bear his mild yoke, they serve him best. His state
>
> Is kingly. Thousands at his bidding speed
>
> And post o'er land and ocean without rest:
>
> They also serve who only stand and wait'.

The first line contains a pun at the end; the word *spent* means both 'spent' in the sense of spending time, and also 'spent' in the sense of an energy or resource that has been used up.

Milton is saying he is worried his blindness makes him useless and unable to serve God. Milton believed that his lot in life was to work hard at his writing and to offer his writing to the world for the glory of God. This sounds like a pious aim, but in fact Milton, far from being some old crabbed religious pedant, was profoundly interested in life and people.

In the poem, he's saying that the affliction of his blindness perplexes him because he wonders whether God still demands that people undertake hard, physical work – 'day-labor' – when they don't have any light. This is the meaning of the line, 'Doth God exact day-labor, light denied?'

Milton is then about to 'murmur' his question regarding whether God would be so cruel as to make impossible demands of a blind man, when 'Patience' steps in to stop him. The remainder of the poem is the counsel offered, in effect, by Patience.

First, Patience explains that God doesn't actually *need* anything, with the implication that this is because God (or by extension, whatever the reader understands by the notion of a deity) is complete and perfect as he is and so doesn't require work or talents ('gifts') of any kind. Patience next goes on to argue that those people who are the best servants of God allow their fates to be linked with and even controlled by God, as if they were wearing a yoke. This, Patience explains, means accepting things as they come, especially suffering and misfortune.

Milton, however, doesn't want to make God sound like a slave driver, so God's yoke is called 'mild'. Using his persona of Patience, Milton argues that God, with his kingly status, has an abundance of servants doing his 'bidding' – that is, carrying out missions for God that require light and vision. But kings, by implication, also have people who stand in a state of readiness until their action is needed.

The culmination of Patience's response to the central question of the poem is wonderfully moving. We can be sure that in this imagined response Milton found much consolation, especially in the final, on the face of it simple, even naïve but in fact magnificent line: 'They also serve who only stand and wait'.

'They' are God's angels. What Milton is saying is *not* that there are two distinct orders of angels – one which is busy doing God's bidding and another which has a much quieter life of waiting. Instead, Patience argues that *all* angels are envoys of God and that some are indeed being sent on missions and are extremely active in carrying out God's bidding, while others waiting to be sent can also be seen as heroes or heroines who have not yet made their mark, but shall before long.

Frankie was an extremely busy and active person, but the nature of her heroism was quieter and less active than the kind of busyness which Milton is talking about in his masterly sonnet. Her heroism was of a more static, reactive kind. While she was in no case a passive person, her heroism expressed itself through her ability to, for a long time, 'stand and wait'. As we get to know her better, we see that, in many respects, her heroism frequently consisted simply of saying 'no' when confronted with an enormous pressure to say 'yes'. Because her consistency in saying 'no' had such a beneficial impact on thousands of lives, it is no stretch of the imagination to think of her as an earthly angel; an angel who would stand and wait until her vigorous action was needed.

Frankie was also a loving and devoted mother. Her children Susan and Christine, were born in 1947 and 1949 respectively. The period of Frankie's life when she was a particular heroine for humanity ran from September 1960 to November 1961. Susan and Christine were young teenagers at the time. Christine told us that she remembers none of the specific work-related matters being discussed by her mother and father at the dinner table during that period:

> Susan and I were very much engrossed in our own thoughts and our own lives at that time, and while we enjoyed Mum and Dad's dinners, we didn't pay much attention to what they were saying over the dinner table.

Frankie and her husband, Dr Fremont Ellis Kelsey – generally known within his family and by his friends as 'Ellis', though some of his close friends called him 'Kelse' – were in similar professions and, as Frankie herself often commented, were an excellent team. They didn't both work at the FDA, but they talked about their work, and they were mutually supportive. All the evidence is that their marriage was highly successful.

Frankie loved being a mother. It's hard to assess how important her mothering skills were to her viewpoint, although in researching her life, one sometimes confronts little gems of highly pertinent insight: for instance, in a letter to one of her friends, Frankie casually remarks that during her own pregnancies, she was even reluctant to have an influenza jab. It's clear that Frankie's reluctance here stemmed from her fear that even such a routine treatment could have a negative effect on her unborn child. Perhaps this chance remark of Frankie's provides some vital insight into why she was so conscientious in her work at the FDA. After all, a mother is bound to be especially conscious of the hazards to her unborn child. Even a full six months before the ghastly truth about thalidomide broke, Frankie – a scientist and a mother too – was deeply suspicious of the possible harm the drug could cause to unborn children.

Frankie was the relatively junior official at the FDA responsible for deciding whether the FDA should allow an application to permit thalidomide to be marketed in the United States. Almost from the start, she was wary of the application. She found that, administratively, the application was of poor quality and did not conform to the FDA's protocols and requirements. This wariness became an antipathy when Frankie discovered that many adult patients who had taken thalidomide in countries where it was permitted had developed a condition called peripheral neuritis – a painful tingling of the extremities that didn't necessarily stop when the patient discontinued thalidomide.

Buried in the Frances Kelsey archive at the Library of Congress in Washington, D.C., there is a memo, handwritten by Frankie, which proves that she instinctively felt that thalidomide might also represent a threat to the unborn. The memo relates to a telephone conversation between Frankie and Dr Joseph Murray, the representative liaising with Frankie from Merrell, the organization trying to get her to approve the drug. While the memo is not dated, the phone call she references took place in the summer of 1961.

Murray of Merrell called to try and get a deadline set for release of Kevadon. I explained I was concerned about the use of the drug in pregnancy because of the possible effect on a fetus and the lack of mention of objective findings in peripheral neuritis. He [Murray] wondered if he could record changes by phone and then print up the brochures for the October deadline (to get product on market by Christmas) or bring them in and have me okay them. I said neither would be acceptable as misunderstandings inevitably result and that he should submit the materials through the usual channels. I said we would get to it as soon as possible but could give no definite commitment.

Asked in later life by an interviewer if she had any memory of when she first became worried that thalidomide might injure the fetus in the womb, Frankie, remembering a meeting that occurred on 11 May 1961, said:

I do recall an occasion when the company [Merrell] representatives stated that since the drug [thalidomide] had been used so widely in Europe in the past few years, if it had a toxic effect on the fetus, it would have been detected. I clearly remember asking them if they could document one hundred cases in which the drug had been used throughout pregnancy. They said that they could not. In light of current information on the detection of most teratogens, this was a woefully inadequate number, but thalidomide is such a potent teratogen that it could have been picked up with even fewer subjects, as was subsequently demonstrated by Dr. McBride.

We look at the vital work of Dr William McBride in Chapter 12. Frankie also comments:

My own recollection is that the question of safety in pregnancy was discussed in-house prior to this meeting, when the report of peripheral neuritis led to a concern about chronic toxicity. The new drug application (NDA) did contain a study of the use of the drug for insomnia in the third trimester of pregnancy, and the labeling included this use, but since the peripheral neuritis was associated with prolonged use of the drug, absence of ill effects [after a] three-month exposure was not sufficiently reassuring. I doubt anyone foresaw that a single dose of this drug at the appropriate time in early pregnancy could have such devastating effects. [The parentheses are Frankie's.]

Perhaps not, but Frankie certainly considered that repeated doses might.

Every woman who became a mother in the United States in the early 1960s, and the descendants of those mothers, and anyone who was born in 1960, 1961 or 1962 in the United States, owes Frances Kelsey an enormous debt. Frances was the only public servant, the only drug assessment official in the whole world, who had an instinctive feeling that thalidomide was not to be trusted. The selfishness, arrogance, stupidity, short-sightedness and sexism of several pharmaceutical company business executives, who should have known better, came appallingly close to causing a medical disaster of unimaginable proportions in the United States.

But as things turned out, they were no match for our heroine.

As if blessed by the fates for what she did for America's children, and so also for America, Frances enjoyed a long life. She was born on Friday, 24 July 1914, and lived until another Friday, more than 101 years later, 7 August 2015.

1

AGNES DONNELLON'S
NEW BABY

A photograph on the Facebook wall of Kevin Donnellon, who was born on Tuesday, 28 November 1961, at Walton Hospital near Liverpool in north-west England, shows him taking his daughter Daisy for a walk. These days Kevin prefers to be called Kev. A handsome fellow with stubble and an impressive wide-brimmed black top hat, he looks jaunty and happy in the photo. Daisy, who was five years old when the photo was taken, has just been eating candy and is wiping her mouth with the back of her hand. In many ways, they are like any other father and daughter going for a walk on a sunny spring afternoon.

Except that Kev can't walk and never has been able to. In the photograph, Kev proceeds down the road in his powered wheelchair, and Daisy stands on the wheelchair behind him, hitching a ride.

Today, Kev is a cheerful, witty, ebullient fellow with a loving and devoted able-bodied wife, Angela, who gave birth to the Donnellons' second child, Ollie, in August 2016.

Kev can't walk because, when he was born – in addition to the fact that he was deaf in his right ear – the long bones in his arms and legs hadn't developed. This was due to his mother, Agnes, having taken, over several days, five tablets of a medicine branded Distaval, which was really a drug called thalidomide. Agnes started taking it soon after she knew she was expecting a baby, because she was suffering from morning sickness.

Kev's condition is known in the medical profession as 'phocomelia'. It derives from the Ancient Greek words *phoke* ('seal') and *melos* ('limb'), and so in effect describes children born with this condition as 'seal-limbed'. This cold medical designation is not, of course, much help to the people who live their lives suffering from this problem.

Normally, phocomelia occurs in about one in every two million births. Most doctors never see a single case in their entire careers. But in the late 1950s and early 1960s, thalidomide led to a horrible epidemic of phocomelia in every country where the drug was sold, until the reason for the epidemic finally dawned on doctors and pharmacologists around the world.

One reason why it took so long to determine that thalidomide was the cause of these appalling deformities was that the drug was branded under so many aliases: Distaval in the UK and Contergan in West Germany, to name only two. In the United States, the intention was to use the brand name Kevadon: it was a bizarre coincidence that the US brand name contained the first name and the first three letters of the surname of a man who was to become one of the highest-profile casualties of thalidomide in the UK.

Kev Donnellon is two feet six inches tall. On his right shoulder he has a hand consisting of three fingers. Attached to them is a tiny useless digit he cannot move. On his left shoulder he has a hand consisting of just two fingers. Attached to the bottom of his trunk are no legs at all. Instead, two perfectly formed feet, each with one big toe and four small ones, grow directly out of his trunk. When Kev was born, his feet were bent upwards, with the heels resting on the floor when he was sitting upright. Kev has become adept at using his feet. He can pick things up with his right foot and even draw with it.

Agnes Donnellon takes up the story. She related it to the makers of a *World in Action* British television documentary about Kev first broadcast in 1971. Several successive episodes were made about Kev as he grew up.

On camera, in that first episode, Agnes explained what had happened late in the evening of Tuesday, 28 November 1961, a few hours after her son was born at Walton Hospital:

A sister came round to the ward at about eleven o'clock in the evening. I thought it was very odd when she came over to my bed and she asked me, did I smoke? I thought it was very strange for her to ask me that at that hour of the night. I said yes I did, and she gave me a cigarette, which I practically choked on, and then she said 'How do you feel?' ... I said, 'Oh, fine, I think.' Then she said, 'I'm terribly sorry, but I have to tell you that you have a little boy, he has a lovely face ... ' – which he had – 'but he's got very tiny arms and legs.'

Of course I looked at her. I thought she meant they were perfect arms and legs, but that maybe he was a midget. I said, 'Oh.' I didn't really know what else to say ... I couldn't really imagine he was like he was. It's just that she said small arms and legs and then she gave me a sleeping tablet, and that was it ... When I woke up the next morning, I thought I had dreamed all this, and I couldn't imagine what she meant.

Anyway, the doctors came the next day to tell me exactly what was the matter with him, which was he had no arms or legs, but two fingers on the left shoulder and three little fingers on his right shoulder, with two little feet attached to his bottom. They asked me would I like to see him, but I didn't feel I was fit enough then anyway, and I don't think I really wanted to see him at the time.

Agnes Donnellon continues:

Of course I used to ask about [how] the baby was, and they used to say he was doing fine, but they didn't really hold much hope of him living anyway, because they thought he would have about three months to live at the most. So just before I was due to come out of hospital – it was nearly Christmas – they asked me if I would like to see him, so I thought I would anyway. So I went down in a wheelchair to have a look at him ... They just took the bedclothes back, and then of course I realized, you know, what I had imagined, but he was worse than what I had imagined. It was a terrible shock, of course. I came out of there and collapsed.

A nurse came over to me and said, 'I wouldn't take him home because you couldn't possibly look after him. I would advise you to leave him here and just go home to your family.' Well, after she said that, with me having four children, my mother instinct sort of came up ... I didn't think she had any right to tell me what to do with my child, so I got in a temper. 'No,' I said, 'I'll take him home. I want to take him home even if he's only going to have three months to live because, after all, he's my son.'

I had four other children, so why should he be treated any differently? So we brought him home.

The story of thalidomide changed forever how the world saw medicine. The story is also a painful example of corporate greed at its worst. When the truth about what thalidomide could do to the unborn baby broke, the name of the drug became a word that terrified pregnant women outside the United States, many of whom – sometimes, tragically, with justification – feared that they had taken thalidomide in the early stages of their pregnancy to counteract morning sickness.

In the countries where the drug was allowed to be marketed, the disaster was compounded by the drug corporations' subsequent haughty indifference to compensating the legion of thalidomide-disabled children. Eventually, compensation was finally paid in some countries, although grudgingly, and in several other countries it wasn't paid at all. The drug companies who had sold thalidomide often claimed that what happened was an accident for which they were not responsible, which was a preposterous argument.

In Britain, for example, only a national campaign by *The Sunday Times* in the 1960s, initiated by the editor Harold 'Harry' Evans (now Sir Harry) followed by a nationwide customer boycott of the Distillers Company's products, forced the corporation to pay compensation to Distaval's victims. In several countries affected by thalidomide there has never been a payout for thalidomide victims at all. In Spain compensation was not awarded until 2013, following a ruling against the German manufacturers.

Other brand names used around the world for thalidomide – which was so potent a teratogenic agent (that is, interfere with the development of the embryo and cause malformation) in humans that it could cause embryonic deformities even if a pregnant mother took only one tablet – included the almost deliberately sinister CC47, and also Actimid, Asmadion, Calmorex, Corona-Robetin, Gastrinide, ImiD 3, Imidene, Profarmil, Quetimid, Quietoplex, Sedimide, Sediserpil, Sedoval K-17, Theophyl-Choline, Ulcerfen, Valip, Softenon, Thalomid, Immunoprin, Talidex, Talizer and Neurosedyn.

According to Dr John Swann of the FDA, there were eighty-nine different brand names for thalidomide worldwide. The drug had far more aliases than any double agent, yet behind its sinister mask, the active ingredient was always the same. When the real side effects of the drug gradually started to become clear, considerable delay in identifying the culprit was caused by the fact that thalidomide had been sold under so many different pseudonyms around the world.

Globally, in the late 1950s and early 1960s, about 100,000 unborn babies – the actual number will never be known for certain – were affected by thalidomide. About half of these died in the womb or a few days after being born. Worldwide, about 50,000 children were born with defects attributable to thalidomide. We estimate that if the drug had been approved by Frankie for distribution, at least another 100,000 thalidomide-affected children would have been born in the United States, and that half as many again would have died.

The devastating effect on these children's families can be imagined only too easily. In many respects, Agnes Donnellon's response was comparatively mild. Many parents abandoned their thalidomide-affected babies completely, left them in institutions, and made only occasional visits – or worse, never tried to see them again. Another factor which made this even more difficult for the families was that thalidomide babies were born for up to five years before the cause was known for certain. Parents had no idea whatsoever what had gone wrong.

Mothers and fathers – mothers especially – blamed themselves for what had happened. Once the cause was known, parents felt even guiltier than they already did about what had happened to their child. Many families split up as a result of the stress, misery and guilt, and there were suicides among fathers as well as mothers. All were traumatized for years; many never recovered.

Despite Frankie's intervention, it is not the case that there were no victims of thalidomide at all in the United States. There were a total of seventeen victims, not due in any way to Frankie being less than diligent in her work but to the fact that, in the early 1960s, bizarrely enough, pharmaceutical companies were allowed to distribute untested drugs to doctors so that the doctors could try them out.

Each one of those seventeen cases of thalidomide in the United States was a disaster, just as every other case was anywhere in the world. Yet, without Dr Kelsey, the thalidomide tragedy in the United States would have been exponentially greater than what it was.

There is no safe way of testing a drug to see if it damages the unborn child. It's not as if there is some spectrum of chemical formulae within which a drug is likely to cause teratogenic effects. Even now, the mechanisms which lead some drugs to cause damage to unborn children aren't fully understood. But the natural processes that must occur in order for a fertilized egg to divide sufficient times and develop so that, nine months later, it becomes a fully developed baby are of such complexity that they defy human imagination. It's not surprising that many artificial compounds – as well as some natural ones – can negatively interfere with the process. Today the concern for possible damage to an unborn child is, quite reasonably, so great that during pregnancy mothers are advised to avoid any medicine at all except what is absolutely essential, and the only medicines that can be safely given during pregnancy are those which anecdotally have shown themselves to be safe.

This approach to medicine and pregnant women is a relatively recent development in the medical industry. In the past, which tragically includes the early 1960s, there was less concern for the effect which artificial substances might have on the unborn child.

This was partly because the idea that drugs could cross the placental barrier – the barrier through which substances, such as nutrients and oxygen, are transferred between the mother and the unborn child – was a relatively new idea, even though it has been known since the nineteenth century that an alcoholic woman could give birth to a malformed child.

The situation wasn't helped by the way women were seen in the 1950s, 1960s, and even well into the 1970s. It was a widespread notion, at the time, that women were inferior to men. Men liked to think that they knew better in all matters, and that women should listen to them and be guided by them. This extended to topics pertaining to women's health.

Sadly, even today, this notion hasn't entirely disappeared. Recent research shows that, in hospitals, women's physical pain is taken much less seriously than men's (particularly when male doctors are involved). As a result, severe chronic conditions are significantly more often misdiagnosed in women: their symptoms, no matter how serious, tend to be dismissed as 'emotional symptoms'.

It may seem a far-fetched hypothesis that the way women were seen at the time would have had an impact on how the thalidomide disaster unfolded, but it isn't. If you look, for example, at television advertisements from the 1960s – and from the 1970s, and even later – for washing machines, the scientific-looking man, often wearing the white coat of the scientist, is contrasted with housewives portrayed as, at best, ignorant of the best laundry detergent to use and, at worst, just ignorant period. These ludicrous ads were strangely popular with women as well as men.

We even find evidence of this attitude in the most unexpected places, such as the otherwise excellent movie *The Sound of Music* released in 1965. A movie that has become iconic, it is about the effects on a repressed Austrian family of a life-loving and rather erratic governess, Maria, famously played by Julie Andrews. The first part of the movie, up to the point where Maria gets married, shows with great emotional conviction and many wonderful songs, how Maria changes the lives of the children and their father, Baron von Trapp. Maria's infectious enthusiasm for life, for music, and for communicating her wonder to the children fills the screen and our hearts.

What is curious about the second part of the film is that, while it remains dramatic, Maria as a character is treated very differently. After she falls in love and then marries the baron, when they return from their month-long honeymoon, Maria is a completely different person. She is quieter, more thoughtful, less impulsive, less imaginative, and less romantic.

There is a clear implication – although probably not intended consciously by the screenwriter and filmmakers – that Maria has been 'tamed' by being married and sexually possessed by the baron. Again, this is a subtext to the film that, while not explored consciously in the story, is inescapable nonetheless, especially to the modern viewer. This subtext says a great deal about how women were seen in relation to men in the 1960s.

Despite the apparently modern impact of the 1960s, whose music and films (not including *The Sound of Music*) were deliberately provocative in terms of their sexuality and storyline, that decade was still plagued by an extremely conservative mindset as far as the role of women in society was concerned. Women were often seen as second-class human beings. We're not suggesting that if there had not been this attitude to women in the 1960s, the thalidomide disaster would never have happened; that would be pushing the point too far. Ultimately, the disaster was caused by poor and, in some cases, ineffective drug regulation, and by the sheer ignorance of the danger which an unknown molecular compound could present when given to a pregnant woman.

All the same, without this stigmatization of women in the 1960s as a kind of secondary citizen, somebody, somewhere along the line, might surely have bothered to pay more attention – and pay attention more urgently – to the reasons for the otherwise inexplicable epidemic of deformed children that flourished in a nightmarish way from the late 1950s until the middle of 1962, by which time thalidomide had been banned worldwide.

Kev Donnellon was born the very week Distaval was withdrawn from the UK market. The entire time he was gestating, a debate – or more accurately, a battle of letters and phone calls – was taking place 3,500 miles away, in the United States, between a particularly profit-obsessed pharmaceutical company called Wm. S. Merrell, later renamed Richardson-Merrell, and referred to mostly in the rest of this book simply as 'Merrell', and 47-year-old Dr Kelsey, Canadian-born but by then a United States citizen. The debate centered on whether Merrell would be allowed to distribute in the US 10 million tablets of Kevadon, containing the same active ingredient that Distaval did. Frankie repeatedly questioned the validity and thoroughness of the new drug application (NDA) Merrell had submitted for Kevadon.

The same week Kev was born, the terrible truth about what thalidomide did to unborn children finally broke around the world. Merrell, with its tail between its legs, would shortly withdraw its application and try to pretend that its months of aggressively trying to browbeat Frankie into agreeing to its proposal hadn't actually happened.

First manufactured in West Germany in the early 1950s, thalidomide's earliest victim was a West German baby girl born on Christmas Day 1956. She was the daughter of an executive of Chemie Grünenthal, the very company that had created the drug. The executive had taken some of the drug home to give to his wife to help combat her morning sickness.

The executive and his wife had no idea what might have caused their daughter's disability – she was reported to have been born 'without ears'. We have not been able to ascertain, despite strenuous research, what the precise nature of this disability was – whether it meant that the baby was born without external ears or without any inner ear at all. What is clear, however, is that for the parents, what happened came completely out of the blue, and this was always a fundamental and traumatizing problem with thalidomide.

At the time, no connection was made between the girl's mother taking thalidomide and the girl's congenital problems. Indeed, no definite connection would be made between thalidomide and congenital deformities for almost another five years, during which time a growing epidemic of deformed babies born in all the countries where thalidomide had been approved for sale became one of the great medical mysteries of the late 1950s and early 1960s, until finally the shocking truth emerged.

Thalidomide, however it was branded, was essentially a vile toxin that should never have been given to pregnant women. Yet soon after thalidomide was launched to the consumer market in West Germany, it was specifically marketed as a sedative and aid to help pregnant women cope with ailments such as morning sickness. It was indeed a powerful remedy against morning sickness, an extremely unpleasant condition for pregnant women.

Unfortunately, while thalidomide did help women with morning sickness, the drug also had a disastrous effect on the unborn child if taken during the first forty days of pregnancy. Depending on when the drug was taken during that time, the tiny growing fetus suffered damage to most parts of its body.

Thalidomide had its devastating impact on embryos who were exposed to it between the twentieth and forty-second day after conception. After that, the developing child – which, by the forty-second day, had the beginnings of a skeleton, a tiny brain that was starting to coordinate movement of muscles and organs, rudimentary reflex responses, a formed jaw with teeth and taste buds, and the outset of fingers and toes – had enough strength to resist the effects of the toxin. The worst of the damage happened when the exposure to thalidomide took place between the twentieth and twenty-eighth day after conception.

When taken in the twentieth day of pregnancy, thalidomide caused central brain damage. On the twenty-first day of pregnancy, it would damage the eyes; on the twenty-second, the face and ears; on the twenty-fourth, the arms; and leg damage would occur if it was taken up to day twenty-eight. Nature's timetable for building a new life is sensitive clockwork.

Kev Donnellon explains:

My favorite way of moving is a sort of sideways hopping. This puts more pressure on my right heel, and consequently I always wear out my trousers in the same position, where the right heel sits. I've developed thicker skin on the underside of my trunk. I can move on a carpet, and on grass and pavements as well. You might imagine it wouldn't be too comfortable moving along a pavement because it's so rough, but actually it's not too bad.

When Kev and Angela's daughter Daisy started preschool, she asked her mother, 'Why does Daddy have a wheelchair?' Daisy was, obviously, used to seeing this wheelchair. It had become such a natural part of her daily life that it hadn't seemed particularly strange to her until she noticed that the other kids' parents at her school didn't have wheelchairs.

Angela and Kev had, in fact, explained the situation to Daisy when Daisy was much younger: they told her Daddy was the way he was because of a 'bad pill' Grandma took. But it had been some years ago when Angela and Kev explained this to Daisy and she hadn't remembered. So Angela gently explained again.

Despite the physical limitations Kev faces, he has had an extremely full life. He's even writing his memoirs, which he's calling, appropriately enough, *Looking Up*. It has its raunchy moments. Before Kev met Angela, he had a varied and adventurous personal life – his first proper relationship was with a lady nurse at a hostel where he was living when he was twenty-two, and in the three decades before he met Angela he had many other relationships. Kev has a handsome face, an affable personality, a gentle wit, and, far from being resentful about his physical situation, he says, 'I'm completely happy nowadays in my own skin; I'm happy about who I am.' He is indeed a happy man, husband, and father. Thalidomide deformities aren't passed on in genes: Daisy and Ollie have no physical limitations apart from being young, and of course they'll grow out of that.

As Kev says, he's one of the lucky ones. For every thalidomide victim who managed to build a good and happy life, there were hundreds who lived short, blighted and painful lives, rejected by their families and growing up in institutions that, for all the efforts of the staff who worked there, were never homes.

Today, the majority of people affected by thalidomide are middle-aged. They are often plagued by persistent, even constant, pain. On top of all the practical problems of their disability, many struggle with depression and financial insecurity. Some have run out of compensation money, and medical equipment is expensive.

However, it's also true that many 'thalidomiders' – a description people affected by thalidomide regard as a respectful generic name – have enjoyed career success in a wide range of fields, including music, writing and inspirational speaking. Others, though, lead limited, unhappy and lonely lives.

The plight of many children affected by thalidomide was made worse because they were growing up at a time when the disabled were regarded as freaks and even as a menace to society. With very limited understanding of the emotional and psychological needs of the disabled, many were forced to wear clumsy, ridiculously heavy artificial limbs, which they hated.

Here's what Louise Medus-Mansell – born, like Kev Donnellon, without arms and legs – writes about her artificial limbs in her life story, *No Hand to Hold and No Legs to Dance On* (2009):

We had to wear the legs from seven thirty in the morning until four in the afternoon on a school day and from seven thirty until twelve on a Sunday. The arms were worn for some classes and some lunches. Saturday we didn't have to wear them at all. We all became quite professional at using them, but none of us liked wearing them, and not just because of the weight. When we had our legs and our arms on we looked like Robocop (or, in today's terms, Transformers). But the arms would dig into me. Every time I moved my hand, I heard *hss, hss* from the gas and water power system, and they were forever going wrong. I felt more disabled in them than I did without.

Louise's book is essential reading for anyone who wants to know more about the effects of thalidomide on a high-spirited, highly intelligent and sensitive young woman. Louise often mentions the kind of casual injustices and cruelties that the disabled endure simply because people are not caring for them properly, or don't care enough about the things they care about:

> Until that summer I had two terrapins, Tom and Tabitha. Tabitha died when I was away on holiday because you are supposed to put olive oil on their shells and turn on the heat lamp. No one had done it, nor had they fed them, so Tabitha had expired and Tom had eaten her.

That same summer, Louise spent two nights living on the streets of London in her wheelchair because there was nowhere else for her to go. Louise's brief but hellish period of homelessness began in October 1979, when she was seventeen, because the place she was living – the Star Centre – had closed and she had to find somewhere to go for ten days. Louise could have avoided her homeless experience because the Thalidomide Trust – a London-based charity that cared for thalidomide victims – was willing to book her a hotel and pay the bill. But Louise felt, not unreasonably, that at age 17, she could look after herself. She thought she had enough money to pay for her own accommodation and the Thalidomide Trust could in due course refund the money into her post office bank account.

Unfortunately however, in those days the British post office bank account was fairly primeval in the way it worked. If you made more than a small number of withdrawals in a week or if there were any mistakes in the account which had to be rectified, the bank book, which was the only way of you had access to your money, had to be sent to the head office. You had no further access to your money while the book was away. In Louise's case there had been a mistake with her account, and she was only able to withdraw £15, which was not enough for her to live on in London. Ironically, Louise was at the time only a short distance away from where her father worked – he owned an art gallery – but as she explains:

> My pride refused to let me go there ... and confess that I'd made a mess of my first trip away on my own. So I just trundled around London, sleeping for two nights on the streets in my wheelchair.

So began Louise's horrific two days living on the streets in her wheelchair. Louise (who is a friend of Kev Donnellon) was badly affected by thalidomide and has very short arms and very short, distorted legs, but her steely determination and energy led her to become a contented mother with happy and healthy children. But that was later. For the moment, at seventeen, on a cold October night, she only had fifteen pounds and nowhere to stay. As she explains:

> I had paid the hotel on arrival for Friday, Saturday, and Sunday, and when Monday came I had to pay for Monday night, Tuesday, and Wednesday, so I went to the nearest post office and gave them my book. The system was then that if they made a mistake, they had to send the book to Glasgow to get it rectified, and you had to wait for three days for it to come back ... This left me in a bit of a fix, to put it mildly. I went back to the hotel and told them what had happened, and they said there was not a lot they could do.

They agreed to keep my stuff for me, so I had an extra-big breakfast, as much as I could stuff inside me, and off I toddled for an enjoyable day at the Tate Gallery. Come the night I had absolutely nowhere to go. I rang the Thalidomide Trust, who told me to go back to the hotel and phone them from there, but, being seventeen, I was too proud to turn up there again without the money to pay ... .

I budgeted for fifteen pounds so I could buy drinks and something to eat, but I quickly ran out, and I ended up starving. You use up an awful lot of calories pushing yourself around, especially when it turns chilly. By the third day my hunger pangs were truly painful. I lost a lot of weight.

I only had a bomber jacket, but luckily it wasn't too cold. I hung around the streets nearest the hotel, hiding in doorways. I made sure I went in the streets where no one else was and looked for a warm corner or a shop window. If anyone came, I waited until they had taken four or five steps past me, then I moved on. It was not so bad because in London you can stay in an [art] gallery or somewhere until six, [and] then, by the time you have had something to eat – though I didn't have enough cash for a proper meal – and go to the loo and mess around in there for an hour or so, most of the evening has gone by.

People don't start getting suspicious about why a limbless person is out on the street in a wheelchair until one or two a.m. Then you have to hide away and be ready to move on until six a.m. when London starts coming to life again and you are no longer conspicuous.

Louise adds:

At nine a.m. on the Wednesday, I turned up at the post office, but my book had not arrived. That was a very bad moment, as I had been so looking forward to breakfast. I had to go back in the afternoon for the second post, and luckily the book was there. I took out fifty pounds, returned to the hotel, paid for my room, had a shower and an enormous dinner, watched a movie, [and] went to bed. Simple things like having a pillow to put my head on after two days were absolute bliss.

Looking back I realize it was not a sensible thing to do, as I was incredibly vulnerable. But at the time I felt pleased with myself having survived without asking anyone for help. It's an experience which has always stayed with me, giving me an understanding of homelessness and of hunger which I would not have had otherwise.

Looking back on his life so far, Kev Donnellon, now fifty-six, says:

Being born with problems caused by thalidomide was difficult in so many ways. When you are a little kid, nobody wants to tell you the truth, and anyway you won't be able to understand it. And besides, it's too horrible to think about, really, that your mother took a drug just because she didn't want to suffer morning sickness, and it ended up damaging you when you were just a clump of cells in your mother's womb, and it meant you were never going to have arms or legs. I mean, that's a pretty terrible thing to know, isn't it? It's not surprising that some children with missing limbs due to thalidomide were lied to by their carers and by their parents and were told that their arms and legs would eventually grow. It was as if the carers feared that telling the little children that their limbs would never grow would be too much for the children to bear. Perhaps it was. And when the children also had internal problems caused by thalidomide and were going to die before long anyway, maybe it really was better for them to believe a lie.

The thalidomide disaster was a total nightmare, something that should have stayed in the realms of the dark imagination, rather than being unleashed on the real world. After all, the story of thalidomide sounds like a dystopian nightmare from a dark fairy tale - a story in which a drug, spell, or some other kind of malign influence damages the bodies of children before they are even born, at a time when they are not even aware of what is going on because they are gestating embryos in a place that should be the safest place in the universe: the uterus of a mother. But thalidomide was not a nightmare from the dark imagination. It was – tragically, unfortunately, horrendously – only too real.

Once upon a time, an evil wizard cursed thousands of innocent babies to be born with horrible deformities. That's what this story should have been: a scary tale, the wicked plan of an evil wizard, something trapped in the imaginary world of fiction. It should never have been a piece of real-life, twentieth-century history.

But it was.

The first half of the twentieth century was the most wicked fifty years in human history, with human depravity and evil having plunged to depths unknown even during the reign of the conquerors. For the first time in history, during that time, concentration camps were created, whose sole purpose was to exterminate members of that community. Thankfully the 'sleeping giant of imperilled civilization', in the words of chief prosecutor Robert H. Jackson at the start of the Nuremberg trial on 21 November, 1945, woke out of its benign slumber and destroyed Nazi Germany and the evils that went with it.

By the 1950s, much of the world seemed to be entering a new dawn. Most countries had never been as prosperous as they were. The benefits of a consumer society were filtering down to all echelons of society itself, and there was a sense that science and progress would make the second half of the twentieth century a great improvement on the first half. And science, technology, and the comprehensive benefits to humanity that went with the post–Second World War era generally did lead to a better life than ever before for millions of people.

However, there was a huge – and with hindsight, excessive – belief in what science could achieve. A major reason for the thalidomide disaster was hubris among medical scientists – almost all male – who believed that their knowledge and wisdom were greater and ultimately more important than the age-old miracle of the creation of a new human being.

This disaster only happened because several large pharmaceutical companies, run almost exclusively by men, discounted the possibility that a new drug, designed as a non-toxic tranquilizer and sedative, and making all of them a fortune, might have had a terrible effect upon the unborn child.

David Mason, the brave and resolute father of Louise Medus-Mansell, said after his courageous (and occasionally single-handed) fight for British victims of the drug to be given fair compensation: 'At the end of the day, my daughter Louise still has no legs'.

And yes, even after the story of Frankie's heroism has been told, people afflicted with problems caused by thalidomide will still be burdened by those problems.

But just because a story doesn't have a happy ending doesn't mean that it can't be inspirational. After all, our stories all have, in one sense, an unhappy ending, as our lives don't go on forever. Yet we can still be heroes and heroines in our own way, we can still leave the world a better place than we found it when we were born, and we can also show, in the way we deal with adversity, that we are a species capable of sublimity, magnificence, and glorious collaboration with one another to create a better world and to right wrongs.

In short, the story of thalidomide can make us proud to be human, while simultaneously making us feel embarrassed and ashamed of the potential our species has for folly.

2

THE DOCTOR'S LETTER

Tuesday, 4 April 1961. In a drab, sparsely furnished office of the United States Food and Drug Administration (FDA) in Washington, D.C., Dr Frances Kelsey, aged 46, a physician and pharmacologist, is reading a letter from a United States doctor whose name has been lost to history.

The letter has been written in support of an application William S. Merrell Inc. first submitted to the FDA on Monday, 12 September 1960. The application is for the granting of a license for a new drug, Kevadon, presented by the Merrell corporation as a miracle sedative, without side effects, which can also cure the morning sickness so often suffered by pregnant women. The request is for Kevadon to be made available on a prescription basis to the entire United States.

This is what the unidentified doctor wrote to Frankie on 4 April 1961:

FRANCES O. KELSEY, MD,
Medical Officer, New Drug Branch, Food and Drug Administration, Washington, D.C.

Dear Dr. Kelsey: As one of the investigators working on thalidomide, I was surprised to learn the other day from Dr. Tom Jones of the Wm. S. Merrell Co. that their application to obtain a license to market this drug has been delayed.

I know that you have already been supplied with all the personal data regarding this drug and the various investigations that have been made to its use. At this time I am merely writing to state that in my experience, it is the safest sedative-hypnotic drug with which I've been acquainted. All together I have administered it to over two hundred people without any evidence of serious side effects. As you know, the compound has been available in Germany for about five years and in England for three years. The only serious complication has been peripheral neuritis, which of course is reversible when the drug is stopped. The incidence of this complication is only one thousandth of 1 percent of 100,000 cases. If the drug were to be withheld for this reason alone, one is inclined to think also that many other compounds already on the market including alcohol sold for public consumption should be withdrawn, since the latter certainly produces peripheral neuritis in many more individuals than thalidomide.

I think one practical point concerning this drug should be weighed rather seriously. The ... extremely low toxicity of the drug, which makes it an outstandingly safe medication to be placed in the hands of potentially suicidal patients. In my own practice I have had three patients who took gross overdosages of the medication in suicidal attempts. All of these recovered promptly without any particular effort having to be made to resuscitate them. Had they been in possession of a barbiturate drug, all would probably have succumbed to the effects of their self-administered overdoses. What can be said about suicidal patients can equally be said about children who might possibly find the drug in a household where it has been carelessly placed. As you know, each year many children are victims of barbiturate overdosage after ingesting such medication which they find lying around. In these respects, then, I would consider that Kevadon, though not a drug that is administered to save life, certainly does save lives by virtue of the fact that overdosage, and even massive overdosage, has never been fatal to a human.

I hope that these remarks may be of help to you and I would appreciate any observations you may care to make about the matter. If there is any information which I can give you, on the basis of my own experience, which might help in reaching a decision, please feel free to call upon me. With very best regards, sincerely yours,

[SIGNATURE]

Peripheral neuritis develops when nerves in the body's extremities, such as the hands, feet, and arms, are damaged. The symptoms depend on which nerves are damaged.

The doctor's letter was of course supposed to be a fervent testimonial to the efficacy and safety of Kevadon. If Frances Kelsey had acted on that letter, the medical history of the post-war United States would be very different.

Regarded by many as the first pharmaceutical company in the United States, the Wm. S. Merrell Company was first established in 1828 in Cincinnati, Ohio, by a young pharmacist named William Stanley Merrell. There is perhaps some significance in the first pharmaceutical corporation in the US being founded in Cincinnati, which is often regarded as the very first wholly American city in the United States, the first city that was founded purely by Americans rather than by foreigners and then often renamed.

Merrell himself started out in business as a small retailer of patent medicines. These branded medicines were each supposed to offer some particular benefit, but in those days before drugs were regulated, they were often fairly ineffective, while other medicines contained potent and dangerous ingredients that today are illegal. Generally, it was a time in medical history when many doctors made more money from selling drugs to patients than collecting fees from the patients for improving the patients' health.

Before long, William Merrell started producing his own medicines as well as selling other people's. Many medicines sold at the time derived from dyes. The dye industry set out to make bright and colorful pigments and in order to do so needed to be relatively sophisticated at inorganic and organic chemistry.

Later in the nineteenth century, the German dye industry in particular began to lead the world. This was substantially due to Germany being without foreign colonies of its own, because by the time Germany was united on 21 November 1871 – when Prussia declared the German state and 'Second Reich' – many countries outside Europe had already been seized by other European countries and turned into colonies.

German chemists consequently set out to become extremely adept at developing dyes and related chemicals, frequently by the reverse chemical engineering of coal. There were also vigorous efforts on the part of pharmacists in Germany and other European countries to investigate whether any synthetic dyes had medicinal properties. In the twentieth century these investigations eventually bore fruit with the development of one of the first effective antibiotics – a dye known as Prontosil Red – in 1932 by a research team at the Bayer Laboratories, part of the German conglomerate I.G. Farben (*Farben* is the German word for 'dyes'.)

In 1936, as a young man, Franklin D. Roosevelt II, the son of President F. D. Roosevelt, contracted a streptococcal throat infection and developed life-threatening complications. His successful treatment with Prontosil, the first commercially available sulfonamide drug, meant that a potentially dangerous surgical procedure which the White House medical staff had considered could be avoided. This successful use of Prontosil Red became famous throughout the US, and it was a major factor in heralding the era of antibacterial chemotherapy in the United States.

The German chemical industry took a severe blow in the First World War, when its overseas market for drugs collapsed due to wartime bans. In the Second World War, Germany became notorious for its inhuman uses of drugs such as the chemical Zyklon-B, a form of hydrogen cyanide used in concentration camps to kill millions of innocent people, which was also developed by I.G. Farben in a twisted about-face of its previous benevolent agenda. As for the United States pharmaceutical industry, it only started to achieved world-class status during the Second World War, mainly as a result of its highly successful work on the mass production of penicillin and on its earlier development of the sulfa drugs, a class of antibiotics.

In 1938, the Vick Chemical Company (Vicks) acquired the assets of Wm. S. Merrell, making it a subsidiary of Vicks. At that time Vicks was mainly involved in the manufacture and sale of household medicinal products and cosmetics; perhaps its most famous product is still Vicks VapoRub. Vicks itself could trace its lineage back to 1880, when Lunsford Richardson, a pharmacist in Greensboro, North Carolina, established the company.

The great success of Vicks VapoRub derived largely from the fact that it contained menthol, which at the time was a relatively unknown drug from Japan. Menthol is an organic compound made synthetically or obtained from corn mint, peppermint, or other mint oils. It is a waxy, crystalline substance which acts as a local anaesthetic and also as a 'counterirritant', producing some irritant effects on the body that lead to the reduction of other more serious irritant effects.

In the 1930s, Vicks diversified into the prescription drug business, as the firm had become convinced that a cure for the common cold would soon be found. As this would make products such as Vicks VapoRub either less popular or completely unnecessary, a move into the prescription drug business seemed like a good idea to Vick and led directly to Richardson's acquisition of Wm. S. Merrell.

In 1960, the Vick Chemical Company changed its name to Richardson-Merrell Inc. The company had a proficient distribution system and was developing several drugs it hoped would catapult it into the front rank of pharmaceutical companies (at the time its position on the Fortune 500 list was about 300). One of these drugs was MER/29, an anticholesterol drug that Merrell itself had developed. Another was a drug developed in Germany, but for which Merrell had obtained licensing rights in the United States and Canada. This drug was thalidomide.

Many westerns made in the United States and elsewhere, set in the days of the Old West from about 1870 to 1890, depict a traveling doctor (or quack) who goes around trying to sell some all-purpose medicine to anyone he meets in the Wild West itself. Frequently this medicine is some kind of snake oil. The very phrase *snake oil* has since become synonymous with a drug that falsely claims to be a cure for pretty much any malaise.

In the movie *The Outlaw Josey Wales* (1976), for example, respected for its historical fidelity to the times, a quack doctor trying to sell Josey a particular proprietary potion incites Josey to spit tobacco juice on one of the would-be vendors' shoes. Josey then asks politely whether the chemical in question is any good against stains.

More seriously, in the nineteenth century in the United States, as well as in all countries of the world, there was no effective drug regulation or significant legislation, and many proprietary products were potentially very dangerous.

However, in 1906 the Pure Food and Drug Act came about, in part, because of rising public alarm about inflated health claims for quack medicines. The man who pioneered this new law was one Harvey Wiley. Born in 1844, the son of a farmer, he enlisted with the Union Army in 1864 and subsequently returned to Hanover College, Indiana, where he had previously studied for about a year, and where he had majored in the humanities. Wiley finally graduated in medicine in 1871. A man of wide intellectual gifts, he became a professor of Greek and Latin at Butler College, Indianapolis, from 1868 to 1870. After his graduation, Wiley accepted a position teaching chemistry at Butler, where he taught what was Indiana's first laboratory course in chemistry, starting in 1873. Eventually he took a faculty position in Chemistry in a newly-opened Purdue University in 1874. He was also appointed State Chemist of Indiana.

In 1878, Wiley traveled overseas, attending the lectures of the famous German chemist August Wilhelm von Hofmann, who had discovered several organic compounds deriving from tar, including the extremely useful dye aniline. While living in Germany, Wiley spent a lot of time studying sugar chemistry, and he used this new knowledge when he returned to the United States to help develop a strong domestic sugar industry by finding ways of detecting the adulteration of sugar. Foods were often adulterated in those days, with compounds that varied from harmless ones such as chalk – which, for example, was often added to flour in order to increase its weight – to those that were positively dangerous.

In 1902 Wiley was awarded five thousand dollars by the US Congress to study the effects of the chemical preservatives being used on human food. The US Congress was concerned about the safety of these preservatives, and Wiley's study completely validated this concern. Wiley became an important crusader in support of national food and drug legislation.

At about this time, Wiley became friends with another health campaigner, Alice Lakey, who was born in 1857. She was an activist in the Pure Food Movement, which was highly influential in American society in the first decade of the twentieth century. Alice first became interested in this work in 1896 when she took over the household duties after her mother Emily died. Her father was picky about food, and this led Alice to be interested in just how justified her father's pickiness was.

Alice was a resident of the village of Cranford in New Jersey, and she joined the Cranford Village Improvement Association's Domestic Science Unit. She soon became president of the entire association. As president, on one occasion she invited Harvey Wiley to speak to the association about tainted food. Spurred on by meeting Wiley and hearing him speak, Alice convinced the Cranford Village Improvement Association to petition Congress to enact the Pure Food and Drug Act. She also made strenuous efforts to ask the National Consumers League to support the cause, and the League created an investigation committee to find out about tainted food and the conditions of the workers who were producing it.

This committee eventually became known as the Pure Food Committee, and Alice Lakey was appointed its head in 1905. She and others, including Harvey Wiley, met with President Theodore Roosevelt that year. Roosevelt asked them to present signed letters in support of the Act to

Congress, saying he would then help them to pass the bill. Due to the efforts of Lakey and others, over one million women wrote letters supporting the Act, and in 1906 the Pure Food and Drug Act passed into law.

The Pure Food and Drug Act of 1906 was the first of a series of significant consumer protection laws enacted by US Congress in the twentieth century that led to the creation of the Food and Drug Administration. The Food and Drug Administration itself was formed on 30 June 1906. Agencies that preceded it included the Food, Drug, and Insecticide Administration, which existed from July 1927 to June 1930; the Bureau of Chemistry, which was formed in July 1901 and lasted until 1927; and the Division of Chemistry, which was established in 1862. The FDA operates under the jurisdiction of the federal government of the United States.

The main purpose of the Pure Food and Drug Act was to ban foreign and interstate traffic in adulterated or mislabeled food and drug products. The Act also directed the US Bureau of Chemistry to inspect products and refer offenders to prosecutors. The Act required that certain dangerous active ingredients be listed on the label of a drug's packaging and that drugs not fall outside purity levels established by the United States Pharmacopeia or the National Formulary.

As an example of the Pure Food and Drug Act's provisions, drug labels had to list any of ten ingredients that were deemed 'addictive' or 'dangerous' on the ingredient list if they were present – and could not list them if they were not present. In particular, alcohol, morphine, opium, and cannabis were all included on the list of these addictive or dangerous drugs. While financial penalties under the new law were relatively modest, a provision of the Act allowed government inspectors to seize and destroy merchandise that failed to comply; this was a powerful practical measure and a significant disincentive for manufacturers to continue to produce such merchandise.

The Pure Food and Drug Act of 1906 was largely replaced by the much more comprehensive Food, Drug, and Cosmetic Act of 1938. This set of laws passed by Congress in 1938 gave the US Food and Drug Administration the authority to oversee the safety of food, drugs, medical devices, and cosmetics. The Act has been amended many times since its passage into law: recently requirements about bioterrorism preparations have been added. The long title of the Act was 'To prohibit the movement in interstate commerce of adulterated and misbranded food, drugs, devices, and cosmetics, and for other purposes'.

Between the passage of the Pure Food and Drug Act of 1906 and the new Food, Drug, and Cosmetic Act of 1938, a medical disaster had occurred in 1937 that many believe spurred the passage of the new Act. The tragedy was linked directly to the German discovery in 1932 of the antibacterial qualities of Prontosil Red. The active ingredient in Prontosil Red was a compound known as sulfanilamide, which was adept at fighting streptococcal infections.

This major discovery prompted several leading pharmaceutical companies – including Merck, Squibb, and Eli Lilly – to begin making sulfanilamide drugs. These medicines were mostly formulated as capsules and tablets. However, the S.E. Massengill Company of Bristol, Tennessee, decided that a liquid form of sulfanilamide could also be a best seller, and would be especially attractive to parents wanting to give the benefits of the drug to their children. But the Massengill Company needed to find a way of incorporating sulfanilamide in a solution that could be taken by children.

The chief pharmacist and chemist of Massengill, Harold Watkins, concocted a solution that consisted of 10 per cent sulfanilamide, 72 per cent diethylene glycol, and 16 per cent water. To make this solution palatable, the Massengill Company flavored it with raspberry extract and saccharine. By September 1937, Massengill had distributed 240 gallons of the liquid, branded as Elixir Sulfanilamide, across the United States.

It soon became clear that Elixir Sulfanilamide had a tragic side effect: death. The initial commercial success of the compound was terminally soured by reports of the deaths of six patients in Tulsa, Oklahoma, who had suffered renal failure following treatment with the drug.

At the time, the FDA did not regulate pharmaceutical drug safety and so had no authority to reprimand the Massengill Company. However, the FDA was able to track down and seize bottles of Elixir Sulfanilamide on a technicality – the word *elixir* was a designation reserved for drugs containing ethanol (alcohol). The FDA's action in this respect is considered to have saved as many as four thousand lives.

It did not take long for the FDA to realize what had gone wrong. The main ingredient of Elixir Sulfanilamide, diethylene glycol, is an extremely toxic compound, currently used in antifreeze, and it is now known to cause renal failure and death. Before all the supplies of Elixir Sulfanilamide could be recalled or sequestered, seventy-one adults and thirty-four children died in the autumn of 1937.

We might ask why the Massengill Company would make the decision to concoct a preparation using diethylene glycol in the first place. The answer is that Harold Watkins was completely ignorant of the toxicity of diethylene glycol when he formulated the new product. Even though the first case of a fatality from diethylene glycol had occurred in 1930 and studies had been published in medical journals stating that diethylene glycol could cause kidney damage or failure, its toxicity was not widely known prior to the incident.

The lack of effective international, information-sharing communications facilities, so much part of our daily life today, was a major factor in delaying the spread of vital knowledge that would have stopped the diethylene glycol disaster in its tracks sooner, just as, twenty-three years later, it could have stopped the thalidomide tragedy. At the time, animal testing for pharmaceutical drugs was not required by law, and Massengill performed none. There were no regulations in place regarding pre-market safety testing of new drugs.

Elixir Sulfanilamide was first sold and distributed in September 1937. The first report of a death occurred shortly afterward, on October 11. As we'll see, Frankie was among the people who assisted on the research project verifying that diethylene glycol was responsible for the fatal adverse effect, about two decades before she began working for the FDA.

The owner of the Massengill Company, when pressed to admit some measure of culpability, infamously answered:

> We have been supplying legitimate professional demands and not once could have foreseen the unlooked-for results. I do not feel that there was any responsibility on our part.

Harold Watkins died by what may have been a self-inflicted gunshot wound while awaiting trial. It is not definitely known whether he committed suicide; his wife insisted that he had accidentally shot himself while cleaning his gun, but this seems implausible and suicide is probably a more likely explanation.

A lady wrote at the time to US President Franklin D. Roosevelt and described the death of her daughter:

> The first time I ever had occasion to call in a doctor for Joan [her daughter], she was given Elixir of Sulfanilamide. All that is left to us is the caring for her little grave. Even the memory of her is mixed with sorrow, for we can see her little body tossing to and fro and hear that little voice screaming with pain, and it seems as though [it will] drive me insane ... It is my plea that you will take steps to prevent such sales of drugs that will take little lives and leave such suffering behind and such a bleak outlook on the future as I have tonight.

This letter reminds us, if we need reminding, that drug regulation is not some abstract discipline, but instead exists to stave off potentially prodigious levels of human suffering.

Today, when there is an established precedent for health and safety legislation, it's worth remembering that most regulation was not in place until some disaster, or many disasters, happened and led to the government – in the case of the United States, Congress – deciding that there was no alternative but to implement the legislation.

In any civilized society, there is always going to be a need for strict regulation of new and existing pharmaceutical drugs. The 1938 Food, Drug, and Cosmetic Act required companies to perform safety tests on their proposed new drugs and to submit the data to the FDA before being allowed to market their products. As for the Massengill Company, it paid a minimum fine under provisions of the 1906 Pure Food and Drug Act that prohibited labeling the preparation an elixir if it had no alcohol in it.

Until the 1906 Act, there were few federal laws regulating the content and sale of domestically produced food and pharmaceuticals, the exception being the short-lived Vaccine Act of 1813, passed on 27 February 1813. It was designed to encourage vaccination against smallpox and to make it illegal for fraudulent and contaminated vaccines to be distributed. The Act was repealed in 1822 and the authority to regulate vaccines was given to the state rather than the federal level.

By the early 1950s the manufacture, marketing, and distribution of drugs and food products had been regulated for close to half a century. By 1960 pretty much all developed countries of the world had some form of regulatory authority for supervising decisions relating to whether a drug was safe for use by the public. The tragedy of thalidomide was that it was only in the United States that a regulatory authority looked deeply into the question of whether the drug should be permitted.

Meanwhile, in Europe – particularly Germany and Britain – in the spring of 1961, deformed babies continued to be born, while other babies were inexplicably dying suddenly in the womb, and nobody had any idea why.

3

MEDICAL MIRACLES

The Second World War, which lasted from 1939 to 1945, was as much a battle of rival technologies as a fight between rival nations. The conflict provided each side with the impetus for technological development in order to outwit the other. Technology commonly tends to progress faster during wartime conditions, and while it's unfortunate that humans have frequently needed to engage in mortal combat in order to be at their most ingenious, the war years were replete with a vast range of technological developments, by no means limited to purely military applications.

Among the most important inventions that were made or initiated during the six-year conflict were mass-produced penicillin, the jet engine, nuclear power, radar, synthetic rubber and oil, rocketry, and enormous developments in transportation, shipping, and aviation (including pressurized aircraft cabins). Less high-profile but still extremely important wartime inventions included the dynamo-powered torch and the jerrycan: the latter was personally requested by Hitler and represents one of the few positive Nazi contributions to human civilization.

The Second World War also ushered in an age when people believed technology could achieve pretty much anything. Even by the time the war broke out in September 1939, the preceding century or so had produced an endless stream of what seemed to many people at the time and often still to many of us today technological miracles. Many inventions we usually regard as twentieth-century ones were actually born in the nineteenth century, such as the telephone and the television (including color television). Most of the theoretical background behind the man-powered flight of a heavier-than-air machine – first achieved by the Wright Brothers at Kitty Hawk on 17 December 1903 – was developed during the several decades preceding the flight itself.

In the early years of the twentieth century, medical science, too, had made significant strides. Perhaps the best-known and most dramatic example of this was the successful use of insulin to treat diabetes in 1922 by Canadian doctor Frederick Banting.

Before Banting's momentous discovery, the disease known as diabetes was always fatal when its severity caused the body to completely fail to metabolize glucose from food. This failure was due to certain specialized cell clusters in the pancreas – the Islets of Langerhans – producing none, or much too little, of the fundamental and vital protein insulin.

Prior to the successful isolation of insulin and its production from the pancreases of animals (usually cows), the only way to slow the progress of diabetes was to prescribe a diet so low in carbohydrates that the price patients paid for staving off death for a few months was a slower death by starvation. The alternative was that the patient failed to metabolize the glucose in the carbohydrates and was slowly poisoned by the unmetabolized elements that remained in the blood. At the same time, the patient's body, desperate for energy, slowly consumed its own body fat and even its own organs.

Drawing from his own research and from the work of others before him, Banting reached the inescapable conclusion that the human pancreas produced a particular secretion, which the body used to convert glucose into energy.

Isolating the secretion turned out to be extremely difficult: the pancreas also produces digestive juices, which would dissolve the special secretion before it could be used when Banting tried to obtain it from the pancreases of dogs. But after careful and painstaking experiments using the dog pancreases, Banting discovered that it was possible to tie the pancreas in a way that would prevent the digestive juices from being generated while allowing insulin to be produced. His ingenuity in confirming the existence of this essential protein and making it available for diabetic patients would save millions of lives.

About six years later, on Friday, 28 September 1928, Scottish chemist Alexander Fleming was experimenting with cultures growing in his laboratory at St. Mary's College in London (now part of Imperial College). He discovered that a culture of the bacteria staphylococci, which he'd left in a petri dish by an open window, had been partly killed by a spontaneous fungal infection.

The fungus was subsequently found to be *penicillium notatum* (at first, Fleming incorrectly identified it as a different strain). Fascinated by what had happened, Fleming investigated the phenomenon more closely. Through laborious experiments, he found that the fungus killed a wide variety of bacteria. Penicillin was the world's first comprehensively effective antibiotic. It was not, however, until the Second World War that penicillin became widely available for treating people afflicted with bacterial infections that would otherwise have killed them or damaged their health permanently.

In fact, it's rather surprising that penicillin wasn't discovered sooner than it was. It had been known informally since ancient times that moulds can help cure infections of the skin, and Russian peasants for centuries used warm soil to treat infected wounds. Soil is replete with antibiotic substances; many extremely useful modern antibiotics, including ones given to people who are allergic to penicillin, derive from soil bacteria. In 1640, John Parkinson, the King's herbarian, a sort of proto chief medical officer, suggested the use of mould as a form of treatment in his book *Theatrum Plantarum* (Theater of Plants). In 1870, Sir John Scott Burdon-Sanderson, who lectured at St Mary's Hospital in London from 1854 to 1862, observed that culture fluid covered with mould would produce no bacteria.

So why *wasn't* penicillin discovered sooner? The answer appears to be partly the same as the answer to the question of why the effects of thalidomide on unborn children weren't recognized sooner: no method existed for the easy and rapid sharing of crucial information within the medical profession.

The other part of the answer is that the particular strain of penicillin which had antibacterial effects, while straightforward enough to grow – it's the green mould that sprouts readily after a few days on citrus fruit whose skin has been partly or entirely removed, for example – needs to be considerably concentrated and available in substantial quantities if it is to have a decisively useful antibacterial effect. Also, *penicillium notatum* mould tends too easily to decay into other, useless moulds.

Researchers working at Oxford University in the late 1930s had been able to isolate the penicillin compound and prove conclusively that it could be used to treat deadly infections, but the matter of transforming the spores from kitchen pests to medicinal powerhouses still remained.

It was mostly owing to the achievements of two pioneers – Howard Florey and a colleague of his, Sir Ernst Chain – that penicillin was made with enough purity and in sufficient quantities to become the miracle drug we know today. A technique known as 'deep tank fermentation' finally allowed penicillin to be grown in the quantities required. Fleming, Florey, and Chain were jointly awarded the Nobel Prize for Physiology or Medicine in 1945 for their work, which saved millions of lives in the war and continues to do so today.

The country that pioneered large-scale industrial manufacture of penicillin was the United States. Interestingly, much of the wartime and postwar production of penicillin in the United States derived from a single rotten fruit: a mouldy cantaloupe discovered by accident at a market in

Peoria, Arizona. The cantaloupe had an especially strong and robust strain of *penicillium notatum* growing on it; this mould was used as the basis for much of the penicillin grown in the United States during the war and ever since.

Gradually, as the twentieth century proceeded and medical science became more and more effective, doctors, pharmacists, and the somewhat mysterious organizations that actually *made* medicines acquired a correspondingly high status. As the reassuring belief in the afterlife generally decreased – and as even the most resolute believers certainly wanted to be saved by the medical profession if they became ill, thank you very much – there was a logical, enormous surge in the status of doctors and pharmacists.

It's easy to forget that this was a revolutionary change from the way the medical profession had been seen in the nineteenth century and earlier. Despite the effectiveness of at least some of the drugs dispensed before the start of the twentieth century (though most were little more than placebos), the doctors of the past were frequently regarded with contempt: the medical profession was not usually considered a proper occupation for gentlemen.

Surgeons, for example, practicing in the days before antibiotics and anaesthetics, tended to be assessed not in terms of their patients' survival rate – which was just as well, considering how low it was – but instead according to how quickly they could saw off a limb. The theory was that the more rapidly the limb could be hacked off, the less the patient suffered, though in fact most patients died from shock anyway, if not from infection. This particular aspect of the function of a medical man (and they were always men in those days) was seen as so fundamental that doctors were often nicknamed 'sawbones'.

Yet many doctors of the nineteenth century, often only too aware of how little they could do for their patients, naturally dreamt of pushing back the frontiers of medical knowledge. Here, for example, is George Eliot writing about Dr Tertius Lydgate, one of the major characters in her novel *Middlemarch* (1872):

Perhaps that was a more cheerful time for observers and theorizers than the present; we are apt to think it the finest era of the world when America was beginning to be discovered, when a bold sailor, even if he were wrecked, might alight on a new kingdom; and about 1829 the dark territories of Pathology were a fine America for a spirited young adventurer.

By the end of the Second World War, many new medical horizons had been crossed, and the days when doctors could do little more than show sympathy and prescribe bed rest were long over. The late 1940s and 1950s brought yet more triumphs of medical technology, along with many other forms of technology.

Infant vaccination, too, soon became routine in the developed world and increasingly too in the developing world. The days when parents had little choice but to take for granted that some of their children would most likely die before reaching their teenage years, let alone adulthood, mercifully started to recede.

Another example of medical science triumphing over the random natural cruelty of infectious disease was the widespread introduction, in the United States and beyond, of Jonas Salk's polio vaccine. This massively reduced cases of this dreaded disease throughout the late 1950s and early 1960s. The number of polio cases in the US fell from 35,000 in 1953 to 5,600 in 1957 and down to 161 cases in 1961. It was a great victory over a virus that was a true natural abomination: what science fiction writer would have had the audacity to invent a gastrointestinal virus that only naturally infects humans and that causes, in about 95 per cent of cases, relatively benign symptoms such as headache, a mild fever, and sore throat, but which in the remaining cases accidentally migrates to the central nervous system, where it can destroy vital motor cells at the base of the brain? Virologists have not identified any useful function which this destruction offers even to the *virus*: it is a purely random and disastrous side effect. The Salk vaccine gave babies and children the blessing of a bodily security system that recognized the virus and destroyed it before it could embark on its often-catastrophic mischief.

As an article in *Life* magazine stated in October 1957:

> The power and the pace of technology [has] ... brought man to the brink of
> his greatest technological accomplishments ... Whether we know it or not,
> whether we like it or not, the daily life of each of us is being changed – and
> is destined to be changed far more – by events taking place in laboratories
> and factories around the land.

The same week in October 1957 as this issue of *Life* magazine appeared
on the newsstands, a new 'wonder drug' was introduced on the German
market. It was called Contergan.

4

THE BIRTH OF
THALIDOMIDE

The new drug was indeed seen by many – especially its jubilant manufacturer – as a wonder drug: it promised to bring mankind relief from
anxiety and sleep disturbance, psychological scars born of the Second
World War, combined with a general feeling of anxiety about the threat
of nuclear conflict as the Cold War gathered pace.

In May 1949, occupied Germany had been divided into two parts: West
Germany, founded from the American, British, and French sectors,
which was a market economy; and East Germany, known as the German Democratic Republic (GDR), a communist state with a centrally
planned economy, founded from the Soviet sector.

In one aspect, at least, the planning brought an unexpected benefit: the
regulatory authorities never allowed thalidomide to be sold to the citizens
of the GDR. As Arthur Dämmrich says in *Pharmacopolitics* (2004), his
history of drug regulation in the US and West Germany, the GDR had:

a unique set of political and structural constraints on medicine and a
radically different relationship between the state and civil society.

These differences led Dämmrich to exempt the GDR from his study. West Germany and the GDR were different countries at this point, so it's not surprising that the medical procedures of the GDR didn't extend to West Germany, and vice versa. The GDR's distrust of Western medicine stemming from political factors was fortunate for the babies of East Germany.

The United States had anxieties of its own; its citizens were living in fear of being technologically and militarily overpowered by the Soviet Union. This fear gained a tangible basis when, on 4 October 1957 – three days after thalidomide went on the market in Germany – the Soviet Union launched the first Sputnik satellite, whose beeping radio filled the ears of the world as it circled the earth, in effect making a loud, nagging claim that the Soviet system was better than American capitalism. Nor did things for the United States improve when, in December of that same year, a Vanguard rocket designed to launch the first United States satellite exploded on liftoff. By that point, the Soviet Union was celebrating Sputnik II.

Was the Soviet Union a utopia where the communist system produced more technological advances than capitalism? That was yet another stress-inducing thought for Western minds in general, and American minds in particular.

The 1950s and early 1960s were overshadowed by the very real fear that, before long, capitalism and communism would collide militarily in a Third World War – a global, nuclear war that would make the Second World War look like a mere skirmish.

So in the US and Europe, fifteen years after the war, the minds of millions of people were still traumatized by their memories of terror and grief. They remembered the aerial bombings. They remembered the Nazi V-1 and V-2 rocket attacks in the last few months of the war. They remembered the deaths of their loved ones. Millions of former soldiers had lost limbs in their heroic fight for their country. So too had millions of German soldiers, who were themselves fighting for *their* country. Visiting Germany as a boy of six in 1964 on a summer family holiday,

James still remembers paddling in a swimming pool and seeing men with missing limbs sunbathing beside the pool. In some ways, thalidomide was a nightmarish reenactment in babies of the lost limbs of the war, and it was especially cruel on Germany, which suffered more cases of thalidomide deformities than any other nation (although thalidomide would have caused an even greater disaster in the United States).

During the Second World War, the Allies had dropped more than 2 million tons of bombs on Germany, causing psychological and emotional scars that would plague their victims for the rest of their lives, just as those sent to German extermination camps but had somehow survived the war had also been traumatized.

In Germany itself, the instigator of the Second World War, the closing years of the war had been a living hell. German citizens, no longer protected by the almost completely depleted Luftwaffe, had to deal with Allied bombers flying overhead at will, day and night, devastating major cities and factory towns. Germans went to sleep at night having no confidence that they would be alive in the morning, and thousands weren't. In 1944 and 1945, the Allied ground invasion crushed Germany between two pincers: those of the British and the French in the west, and of the Soviets in the east. Many German citizens fled westward to confront the lesser of two evils.

In August 1945, about 4,000 Berliners died of malnutrition every single day, and half the babies born in Germany that month failed to survive. By the end of 1945, only 12 per cent of the children in Cologne had a weight that was normal for their age, and it was the same story throughout Germany. While US occupying forces in Germany enjoyed a daily ration of 4,200 calories, many Germans were making do with 700 calories per person per day, less than half the amount recommended by the League of Nations in 1936 as the minimum necessary for an adult. In the British zone, the ration dropped to only 400 calories per day – less than the amount of food allocated to the inmates of the Bergen-Belsen concentration camp under the Nazis. Germany was paying the price for insane gothic gamble for world domination and ideology based on government-sponsored extermination of peoples regarded as inferior to Germans.

Not surprisingly, a culture of taking tranquilizers and sleeping pills came to dominate most developed nations in the 1950s. One doctor testified to the United States Congress that 'the people of this nation are being steadily educated by doctors and the drug industry to take a drug whenever they felt anxious about anything.' It's been estimated that, during the 1950s, in Britain, one out of eight National Health Service prescriptions was for sleeping pills.

Many of the tranquilizers were extremely dangerous. Barbiturates were particularly risky. The nature of the chemistry of barbiturates meant that establishing the safe dosage was never easy. In 1955, the United States manufactured almost 4 billion barbiturates, or twenty-six pills for every man, woman, and child in the country. Senator Hubert Humphrey announced that one out of every seven Americans was taking barbiturates.

In June 1956 Aldous Huxley pointed out in an article in *The Sunday Times* that human beings had been taking mind-altering drugs since pre-history, especially alcohol. 'Will the pharmacologist be able to do better than the brewers and distillers?' Huxley wondered, then went on: 'It seems reasonable to suppose it.' He was right. But even though there were a few detractors who pointed out that drugs could be a mixed blessing and could have unpredicted side effects that no one could foresee, the general climate of the culture was that these drugs offered hope for those suffering from the psychological wounds of the age.

By the end of the war, the ravages of bombing and street-by-street, village-by-village, town-by-town, and city-by-city fighting had created a Germany that largely comprised piles of rubble.

Some members of the British government estimated at the time that clearing the rubble away would alone take fifty years. But they had reckoned without the hard work and determination of the Germans, who were about to start building, by peaceful, industrious means, the economic prosperity that the Nazis had failed to achieve by fighting. For the time being, Germany was in a terrible situation. Things gradually improved though, at least in the Allied-controlled part of Germany that was to become West Germany. Under the Marshall Plan, which gave Western Europe a total of $120 billion in current dollar values over four years, the US was able to shower West Germany with aid.

Against this unpromising background, a pharmaceutical corporation was founded, in 1946, by a family called Grünenthal, in an abandoned seventeenth-century copper foundry built out of stone, in the small West German village of Stolberg, near Aachen – a town famous for, among other things, being located on the German border with the Netherlands.

The corporation, named Chemie Grünenthal by its founders, initially set out to produce ointments, cough medicines, disinfectants, and herbal remedies. When Grünenthal started operations on its unusual site, many of the surrounding towns and cities – particularly Düsseldorf, the closest large city – were still shattered by bombing and had not yet been rebuilt.

The new corporation was ambitious. It was the first German pharmaceutical company to supply penicillin to the German market after the Allies lifted the ban on supplying the antibiotic to Germany. By the year 1950, Grünenthal was producing this life-saving antibiotic both in oral and injectable form. Grünenthal achieved much financial success and growth from its launch into the antibiotic market, and its management and research team started trying to make new drugs they could originate themselves.

Grünenthal resolved from the outset to conduct market-driven pharmaceutical research; they weren't remotely interested in dilettante research for its own sake. They wanted to develop drugs that they could sell at a profit to the largest number of doctors in Germany and ideally around the world.

Given the success with penicillin and the dire state of Germany in the years immediately following the war, it's not surprising that one of the main areas of research that interested Germany's pharmaceutical companies generally, and Grünenthal in particular, was developing new antibiotics.

The man who headed Chemie Grünenthal's research and development team was Dr Heinrich Mückter. Two years before he joined Grünenthal, Mückter had been a medical scientist for the army of the Third Reich. By the time the war ended, any work undertaken for the Third Reich was likely to have a stigma attached to it, but as Hitler's regime was the government of Germany for thirteen years (from 30 January 1933, to the German surrender on 7 May 1945), German residents who wanted to work in their own country had little choice but to be employed by the Third Reich or by companies operating under the Third Reich's approval. This, of course, doesn't excuse the abominations many Nazi doctors committed in concentration camps and elsewhere.

Mückter himself had plunged into his Nazi career with considerable enthusiasm. He was Medical Officer (or *Stabsarzt*) to the Superior Command of the German Occupation Forces in the city of Krakow, in Poland. He had the additional title of 'Director for the Institute of Spotted Fever and Virus Research', which sounds like a Nazi euphemism if ever there was one.

In the somber words of Trent Stephens and Rock Brynner, in their book about thalidomide *Dark Remedy* (2000):

> The German army was not renowned for missionary medical work in Poland. Given the role that military medicine played in the objectives and methods of the Nazi occupation of Krakow, one can only presume that Mückter's work there involved the science of killing rather than healing.

Like all Germans who had been involved with the Nazi regime but had been lucky enough to escape prosecution for their wartime acts, Mückter was desperate to start a new career. In his case, it was a new phase of his career, which would free him of the taint with which the fallen bloodthirsty regime had contaminated him.

Within a year in his new job at Grünenthal, Mückter had shown himself a star by managing to produce effective and abundant penicillin from mould cultures. Thus Grünenthal started out by making a useful contribution to German economic resurgence and improving health in Germany at the same time. However, the corporation, aware of how much money there was to be made by producing new drugs that would steal a march on rival pharmaceutical companies around the world, soon became notorious for bringing drugs to market without sufficient testing.

It's difficult to know, even with the hindsight of history, whether this behavior was a cultural leftover from the days of the Third Reich – when the only value that mattered was the necessity of serving Germany's interests, while considerations of morality, compassion or the very sanctity of human rights were deemed unworthy of a thought – or Grünenthal simply got carried away by its enthusiasm to make money and so contribute to Germany's recovery.

In one particularly notorious case, between 1953 and 1954, Grünenthal developed an antibiotic, a variant of Streptomycin, called Supracillin. Streptomycin, while a powerful drug extensively used around the world at the time to treat tuberculosis – the drug is still occasionally used today as an antibiotic and pesticide, but has largely been replaced by other safer and more effective medicines for the treatment of TB – was known to have serious side effects. In particular, it could damage nerves between the inner ear and the brain, resulting, in some cases, in the patient going completely deaf. It could also cause nausea, vomiting, and vertigo.

Grünenthal boldly claimed that its research and development team had shown that Supracillin could completely eliminate the side effects of Streptomycin. Their claims for Supracillin turned out not to be justified: nausea and an upset stomach were common problems associated with taking it. Mückter and his team also produced another antibiotic, branded Pulmo 550, which they went so far as to claim was even better than penicillin. But Grünenthal had ignored reports of Pulmo 550 causing severe side effects, and they lost much credibility in the German pharmaceutical industry for using this antibiotic on people before testing it thoroughly on animals.

It soon became clear to Mückter and to his colleagues at Grünenthal that developing new antibiotics that would have the desired effect without side effects was far from easy. Seeking more profit and less trouble, Grünenthal branched out into researching and developing other kinds of new drugs.

One of the leading members of Mückter's research team was another former Nazi, a charmless character called Wilhelm Kunz. Kunz had his own wartime history, having served as a sergeant, and by all accounts he had the kind of domineering, bossy personality which was more suited to the Nazi epoch than to post-war life.

It's not entirely clear what background Kunz had in the sciences, except that he was certainly not an experienced pharmacist or medical professional. Despite this, and for reasons that are also unclear and that we've been unable to ascertain, he was made the head of chemical research for Grünenthal's research and development team, with a brief to engage in mixing organic compounds to find something with beneficial pharmacological potential; the brief was as general as that. Under their employment contracts, both Mückter and Kunz were entitled to a percentage of profit from any drug they developed that turned out to have commercial potential.

Organic chemistry, which was originally the chemistry of compounds occurring in living things (hence the name 'organic') is the chemistry of the element carbon. Carbon has a property that is close to unique in the table of elements: it is extraordinarily capable of bonding itself to other kinds of atoms, as well as linking up its own atoms into long, complex rings and chains. Many of the resulting compounds are found in the human body and in the bodies of all other living creatures, including plants. While some of these compounds have been successfully synthesized, the vast majority have not.

Organic compounds are much more complex than inorganic compounds. In 1954, there were about a million known carbon-based organic compounds. Today, there are about 10 million, yet that number is only a fraction of the number of compounds that are theoretically possible under standard conditions. For this reason, carbon has often been referred to as the 'king of the elements'.

Essentially, in organic chemistry, every molecule consists of a framework of carbon atoms bonded with other atoms. A crucial issue in organic chemistry is how many bonds each atom in the molecule has. Organic chemicals differ enormously in this respect. Organic synthesis is a special branch of chemical synthesis and is concerned with the construction of organic compounds via organic reactions. The synthesis of organic compounds has developed into one of the most important branches of organic chemistry.

The molecule Kunz developed and subsequently christened 'thalidomide' contains thirteen atoms of carbon (C), with four links that are, in effect, docking stations for other molecules. There are also two atoms of nitrogen (N), with three links each; four atoms of oxygen (O) with two links each; and ten of hydrogen (H) with one bond each. This can be stated as a formula: $C_{13}H_{10}O_4N_2$.

Kunz created the new compound following an experiment he conducted to try to find a simple, inexpensive method for manufacturing antibiotics from peptides, that is, the bonds that hold amino acids together to form biologically active molecules (commonly known as proteins). Even though Mückter and Kunz did not have a good track record of developing antibiotics, they had not completely given up trying to do this. One of the experiments Kunz conducted in his attempt to make antibiotics from peptides was to heat a commercially available chemical with a tongue-twister of a name – phthaloyl isoglutamine – and see what happened. The result was thalidomide. Grünenthal immediately began testing it in an effort to find out if it might have any pharmacological benefits on people.

To those unfamiliar with the operation of the pharmaceutical industry, searching for a new drug by trial and error and then seeing if it has any positive benefits may seem a counter-intuitive, not to say absurd, method of proceeding. Yet this is the usual way in which many drugs that turn out to be beneficial to people are created. It is rarely possible to predict with complete accuracy – or often, with any accuracy at all – the particular effect a new organic chemical might have on human beings. Thalidomide was a terrible example of this.

It is sometimes possible through knowledge of biochemistry to get some idea of whether the drug is likely to be effective therapeutically, but in organic chemistry, the difference between a compound that has great benefits and one that is highly toxic can be a matter of a slight variation in an extremely complex formula. In practice, it is easier to discover a new drug, then find out whether it has any useful applications, than it is to try and develop a molecule that will cure a specific disease.

When the researchers at Grünenthal began testing their new molecule, they soon realized it wasn't effective as an antibiotic, nor did it appear to have any effect on reducing tumors in mice, so it seemed unlikely that it would have an anti-cancer property either.

One positive property which thalidomide *did* seem to have was its failure to kill laboratory rats, no matter how high a dose those rats were given. This feature of thalidomide especially excited Grünenthal. Also, certain members of Kunz's team – in particular a researcher called Herbert Keller – were intrigued by the structure of thalidomide, which reminded Keller of the structure of a barbiturate.

These observations led Keller to hope and believe that thalidomide should have a sedative effect on people. He and his colleagues – especially his superiors, Mückter and Kunz – were excited at the possibility that they might have created a sedative that was not toxic to human beings and could not be used in a suicidal or accidental overdose.

Mückter and Kunz soon became obsessed with the idea that thalidomide was some kind of wonder drug which would sedate people without killing them, no matter how large a dose they took. The tests of thalidomide were extended, showing that very high doses of thalidomide wouldn't kill mice, guinea pigs, rabbits, or dogs either.

There is a mystery about what happened next: the records of the research Grünenthal conducted into thalidomide have largely been lost, either deliberately or accidentally. Needless to say, some skeptics feel that this event was too helpful to Grünenthal to have been an accident.

When the testing of thalidomide's sedative effects proved inconclusive on animals, Grünenthal's next step was to try to see whether it had a sedative effect on people. Instead of conducting a methodical, clinically controlled testing of the drug's effects on human beings, Grünenthal simply distributed free samples of thalidomide for doctors to give their patients, and asked doctors to report back on the effects they observed.

The nightmare, now initiated, proceeded with a kind of ghastly inevitability. These informal tests produced a response from doctors and from patients that exceeded Grünenthal's most optimistic dreams. While thalidomide did not have much of a sedative effect on animals, in human beings it induced a pleasant sleep and radically reduced the incidence of headache and other symptoms of anxiety. Most of the physicians involved in the trials in Germany were highly impressed by thalidomide's pleasant sedative effects on their patients.

There is some evidence that thalidomide may have been developed even earlier than in the 1950s. Although there is strong and abundant evidence that Grünenthal developed it, some researchers believe that it was initially developed during the war by the Nazis – and particularly by a scientist called Otto Ambros, a Nazi war criminal, who was known to have advised Grünenthal in the development of thalidomide. A document found by an Argentinian writer, Carlos de Napoli, implies that the drug was tested in the death camps. De Napoli has evidence that, in November 1944, a document from the German pharmaceutical company I.G. Farben – infamous for developing the deadly Zyklon-B cyanide pellets used in the concentration camps – refers to a substance with the same chemical formula as thalidomide. But Grünenthal denies that the thalidomide formula was developed anywhere other than in its own laboratory. Even if thalidomide was developed during the Second World War, the fact that it was designed to be an antidote for nerve toxins seems to make it unlikely that it would have been used in the death camps, as the Nazis were not very interested in giving people in the death camps antidotes for anything except life.

Whatever the dismal truth about the origins of thalidomide, there is no doubt that Grünenthal launched the drug onto the world. Had Grünenthal really developed a miracle drug? They certainly thought so, especially when further reports from doctors in Germany who had been given free samples revealed that thalidomide was particularly helpful in soothing morning sickness in pregnant women. Mückter, Kunz, Keller and the rest of the Grünenthal drug development team were, not surprisingly, ecstatic.

The results seemed so conclusive that, instead of conducting further detailed tests to look into what side effects the new drug might have, Grünenthal – benefiting from the post-war confusion of Germany, in which the national regulatory framework for new drugs was feeble and did not offer many obstacles to enthusiastic chemists itching to launch their new products on an unsuspecting public – went to market.

On Tuesday, 1 October 1957, thalidomide was released into the West German market as a sedative under the name of Contergan, its first alias.

With hindsight, the decision to launch thalidomide on the German market without testing it for potential effects on the unborn child seems insane, yet one needs to bear two crucial factors in mind.

First, as we've seen, in the 1950s it was still not widely believed even by most doctors that drugs given to pregnant mothers could necessarily cross into the developing baby's circulation, although there should have been an awareness of this: from the nineteenth century at least it had been known that babies of alcoholic mothers could be born with physical and mental abnormalities.

Second, the testing that Grünenthal carried out on rats was not directed at seeing what effect it had on their embryos, but rather on seeing if the rats could be given a fatal overdose, which was difficult to achieve at even the highest realistic overdose limits.

But even if Grünenthal *had* investigated the effect of its drug on unborn rat babies, the results would have been hopelessly misleading. A tragic fact about thalidomide – which only became clear later – is that, for reasons that are still not fully understood, primates are far more susceptible to its teratogenic effects than rats and other animals, which only suffer embryo damage with huge doses of the drug.

In effect, the pregnant women of Germany, and other pregnant women around the world, would, without their knowing it, be used as guinea pigs to see if thalidomide caused birth defects.

In West Germany the new drug didn't even need to be prescribed by a doctor. Grünenthal was so sure of its safety that it successfully lobbied for the drug to be available on an over-the-counter basis. They christened their new drug using the last four letters of their name as the first four letters of the name of the drug. From the outset, Grünenthal put enormous conviction and effort into marketing what would turn out to be – when taken by pregnant women, anyway – one of the most abominable drugs ever developed by human beings.

The notion that German scientists had developed a safe and effective sedative was, naturally enough, a matter of national pride for a country that badly needed to rebuild a positive image of itself.

Grünenthal's marketing campaign for Contergan was successful from the outset. Over the three-year period following the launch of the drug, sales grew steadily. By the start of 1961, thalidomide was easily the best-selling sedative in Germany, selling five times as much as the leading sedative competitor.

Before long, sales of thalidomide represented an astonishing 50 per cent of Grünenthal's total corporate income. Many of the corporation's executives – men who could remember only too well what it was like to be poor and hungry and to have enemy bombers flying overhead – became personally wealthy because of contractual arrangements similar to those that had been extended to Mückter and Kunz. As thalidomide prospered, so did Grünenthal executives.

Grünenthal itself grew dramatically, in harmony with the success of thalidomide. Between 1954 and 1961, Grünenthal increased in size from 400 to 1,300 employees – a growth of over 300 per cent.

By September 1960, thalidomide (as Distaval) had been available in the UK for about a year. The drug was available in most European countries, and also in other more far-flung markets, such as Australia and Japan.

Yet of course the biggest potential market of all for Grünenthal's wonder drug was Britain's wartime ally across the Atlantic Ocean, a nation which, in 1960, had a population of about 181 million, tens of millions of whom were women of child-bearing age who didn't want to suffer the distress and discomfort of morning sickness.

Thalidomide was heading for the United States.

5

THE ADVENT OF
FRANCES OLDHAM

One of the most important sources about Frankie's life is a document entitled *Autobiographical Reflections* (we refer to it here as the 'memoir'), which provides remarkably detailed information about Frankie's life and originates from Frankie herself.

Autobiographical Reflections is not a formal autobiography; it was drawn from several disparate sources. These include oral history interviews conducted with Frankie in 1974, 1991 and 1992; a presentation Frankie made on Founder's Day at St Margaret's School, Duncan, British Columbia, in 1992; and a presentation at Frances Kelsey School, Mill Bay, British Columbia, in 1993. The document, being the work of a US Federal employee, is not subject to US copyright.

At the beginning of her memoir about her life, Frankie recalls receiving in 1987 a letter from an eighth-grade girl at the Jolley School in Vermillion, South Dakota. The school, which still exists today, is located in affluent, palatial surroundings on South University Street, Vermillion.

Frankie says that she remembered the letter for two reasons: first, because she and her family had lived in Vermillion, and her daughters had gone to Jolley School. Second, Frankie recalls that the young correspondent asked her some questions that Frankie didn't feel that she answered very well at the time and so she, Frankie, thought she might weave better answers into her reflections on her life.

The eighth-grader, whose name has apparently not been recorded, had to give a speech at her school about a woman who had forged a successful career in spite of obstacles. The girl, who enterprisingly decided to write to Frankie, told her she had obtained some background information on her from the library. Frankie remarked that the eighth-grader 'seemed to have done a good job'. As Frankie also remembers:

> She asked me for a few more facts, but what drew me up short was when she said: 'But, most of all, perhaps you could describe how hard it was to be a woman studying science and medicine when most of your classmates were men. Perhaps you could also tell me how frustrating it must have been to find work when most people thought a woman should only be a housewife'.

It seems strange to think that there was actually a time, not so long ago, when women were regarded as designed mostly for housework and being a housewife, but that was indeed the case. It's essential to remember that Frankie – as a woman scientist, pharmacologist, and vital part of the regulatory team at the FDA – was, at least when she was locked in conflict with Merrell over the thalidomide NDA, one of very few women to hold such an influential position. Indeed, the fact that Frankie was a woman – in the thinking of people like Murray – was one of the many factors that irked Merrell about her. For them, women belonged in the kitchen, not scuppering Merrell's lucrative plans to sell millions of tablets of their wonder drug in the US.

Frankie goes on to say that, when reflecting on her life and how she got involved in studying drugs, she would give an overview regarding what she might have considered obstacles, but she'd also point out how, for her at least:

Good fortune always seemed to come along at the right moment, just when I thought I was down on my luck. One probably should not tell people to 'trust luck and you will get along in life', but it worked pretty well as far as I was concerned.

Frances Kathleen Oldham was born on Friday, 24 July 1914, at Cobble Hill on Vancouver Island, British Columbia, Canada. Cobble Hill is a small community located about 28 miles north of Victoria in the Cowichan Valley Regional District. It is known for its agricultural surroundings and for Cobble Hill itself, which gave the village its name.

Victoria is the capital city of the Canadian province of British Columbia and is located on the southern tip of Vancouver Island off Canada's Pacific coast. Cobble Hill – sometimes mistakenly referred to as 'Cobble Hill Mountain' – is a major attraction for hikers and outdoor enthusiasts in British Columbia. It is just over eleven hundred feet high and mostly covered in evergreen and maple trees. It has a network of trails and paths running along the hillside in a switchback fashion.

As Frankie recalls:

My father was an officer in the British Army and retired to Canada; that was why I was born in Canada. I was named Frances Oldham and was known as Frankie. Things were somewhat different in those days. The roads were narrow, and we did not get a car until I was nine years old. We were dependent on a horse and buggy to get around. My mother taught my older brother how to read and write, and I just listened in and picked it up. For the next two years we traveled, and I went to schools both in Victoria, British Columbia, and in England.

Frankie's mother, Katherine Booth Stuart, known as Kitty, who lived from 1881 to 1950, was born and raised in Edinburgh, Scotland. Frankie's father, Frank Trevor Oldham (1869–1960) was born in Australia on 9 October 1869, and went to school in England, at Clifton College –

which still exists – in Bristol. He joined the British Royal Field Artillery (RFA) in 1889.

The RFA of the British Army provided close artillery support for the infantry. It was created as a distinct arm of the Royal Regiment of Artillery on 1 July 1899, and was re-amalgamated back into the Regiment proper, along with the Royal Garrison Artillery, in 1924. The RFA was the largest arm of the artillery. It was responsible for the medium-caliber guns and howitzers deployed close to the front line and was reasonably mobile.

The RFA was organized into brigades attached to divisions or higher formations. In his career in the RFA, Frank was mainly stationed in India, except for a short time he spent in China during the Boxer Rebellion. Frank retired in 1910 and traveled to Vancouver Island to buy land and settle there. On the boat as he traveled from India to British Columbia, he met Kitty, and they became engaged. Kitty returned to Scotland while he stayed on Vancouver Island, bought land, and built a house. He then traveled to Edinburgh, where they married.

On 13 May 1996 Frankie wrote a memo to Dr John Swann, giving some detailed information about her father. The parentheses are Frankie's.

My father was very pleased with an American decoration, the Order of the Dragon, which he received. As I recall, it was a medal with a predominantly yellow ribbon, and there was also a dragon-decorated certificate. I remember him saying that at that time the US did not recognize military medals (or [it could] have been that the Boxer Rebellion had not been officially recognized) and that the services somehow issued them independently.

However, a few years ago at the military museum, I saw a display devoted to the Boxer Rebellion that contained the Order of the Dragon medals. The British evidently recognized the medal since he wore it with others on ceremonial occasions. My father was greatly entertained by the fact that two acknowledged experts on military medals stopped and asked him what it was. One of the curious was the Prince of Wales (later, briefly, Edward VIII) about 1920 and the other Prince Philip, husband of Queen Elizabeth II in the 1940s.

My father often spoke of his American companions and particularly of a veterinarian, who was given to extolling the virtues of some liniment, whose name I have unfortunately forgotten, in treating a variety of ailments in both man and beast. He gave me some mementoes of his experiences in China, a bamboo opium pipe, a carved ivory figurine, and a Chinese sword, the blade of which had been seriously distorted by enemy artillery.

Frank and Kitty returned to Canada, where they had a son, Stuart, in 1912, and where Frankie was born on 24 July 1914. When Frankie was born, Frank was 44 years old. In August 1914, Frank decided to come out of retirement, re-enlisted, and went to England for four years. After the war, they had two more children, John and Monica, and enjoyed their retirement years on Vancouver Island.

Christine Kelsey says of Stuart:

Uncle Stuart was born in August 1912 (not sure if August 21 or 22). He left for England to attend Clifton College (same school Grandpa had attended) in about 1927. When we knew him in the 1950s, he was the owner of a sawmill (Pioneer Pete's) in Vernon, British Columbia. He and his wife Molly had two daughters, Marilyn and Nancy, and he died in 1975.

Christine writes this about her maternal grandfather, Frank:

Sue and I remember him very well – our family visited him every summer, ending in the summer of 1960. In 1959, we were all together when the Queen visited Vancouver Island as part of a tour of Canada. He was very proud of his years in the army, and wore all his medals at the local parade for the visiting monarch. Grandpa was particularly pleased when Prince Philip stopped to ask about his medals, and one in particular that Prince Philip had never seen. It was an unusually colorful medal given to Grandpa by the American army, for his service in the Boxer Rebellion. It was also very unusual for the US to give a medal to a member of the British forces.

Like most families, the Oldhams had many legends, some of which were even based on truth. There was a minor but fascinating connection between Frankie's mother and Edward Elgar, the illustrious British composer, who lived from 2 June 1857, to 23 February 1934. Among his best-known compositions are orchestral works including the *Enigma Variations* (1898–1899) and the *Pomp & Circumstance Marches* (1901–1930), concertos for violin and cello, and two symphonies. He also composed choral works, of which perhaps the most famous is *The Dream of Gerontius* (1900).

Elgar is one of the best-loved composers in Britain and is regarded as a quintessential English composer. He was a Roman Catholic, came from extremely humble origins, and married the daughter of a senior British army officer. This may be why Frankie's mother – whose husband was, as we've seen, in the army – met him.

Frankie recalls:

[Seeing a] picture of Edward Elgar ... reminded me of a story my mother told of being seated next to him at a banquet during a musical festival at Norwich.

Our research shows that Elgar had a close friend in Norwich called Walter Hansell, and that Elgar would sometimes stay with Hansell when in the Norwich area, and they would on occasion attend concerts together. It is known that Elgar and Hansell spent time at the Norwich musical festival in 1905. This may have been the festival where Frankie's mother met Elgar, but we've not been able to prove this.

Frankie relates:

Not being particularly musical, she [Frankie's mother] was a bit taken aback when he [Elgar] asked her what she thought of his performance – however, she did say what had impressed her most was how well groomed he was compared to the other performers. To her surprise, he said that was the greatest compliment she could bestow on him. It seems his mother hadn't wanted him to enter the music profession because of her lack of pride in [the] appearance of male musicians. He promised her that that would not be the case with him, and Mother's remarks reassured him that he had lived up to his promise!

On Kitty's side were two models of accomplished women: one of Kitty's sisters was a doctor and another was a lawyer.

Frankie recalls her own childhood education:

I think I was used to being in a class with boys because the first school I started out in, Leinster Preparatory School, a small private school in Shawnigan Lake, British Columbia, was theoretically an all-boys school, and for several terms I was the only girl. Later more girls were present. So I started off in the atmosphere of boys, particularly since I had a brother who was two years older.

The school was run by two Irishmen, a father and son, and there was no grade structure. You worked to the level of your ability and the ability of the teachers. I learned a lot of Latin and some algebra and geometry, but the school was a little weak on things like history, French, and English. The school was in existence for about three years until the Depression, I think, finished it. After a year of private coaching by Margery Gillett, I went off to Victoria to finish up eighth grade at high school.

Frankie's recollections of her childhood are beautifully evoked, especially as she wrote this at least seventy years later. We already might well be tempted to think there is something significant in the way she was brought up with Stuart and the way she followed his lessons and taught herself things and then spent several years at a boys' school as the only girl. It seems indisputable that she gained a confidence in her own abilities, despite being a girl we might facetiously add, and that she felt from the outset that she was just as good as a boy in her studies and intellectual achievements.

Frankie proceeds:

I did get some very important and useful lessons in Cobble Hill while I was still at home. I had painting lessons in a class run by Connie Bonner. We largely painted flowers and birds. I took piano lessons from Mrs Edna Baiss. She was a concert pianist in Ireland before she and her husband James came to British Columbia to run a poultry farm just outside Cobble Hill. I took dancing lessons in the old Wilton Hotel. A series of people ran it, but the person I remember best was a young instructor not much older than myself named Dorothy Bird. The Birds lived at Mill Bay, and she was extremely talented. She went off to study at the Cornish School in Seattle and then to New York.

Frankie also recalls:

The last time I saw her [Dorothy] she was organizing a class in modern dance in the Long Island Public School. In another area, I owe part of my early education to my old friend Jerry Mudge, who taught me how to shoot and fish and, without my parents' knowledge, gave me my first driving lesson.

One yearns for more details of young Frankie being taught how to shoot and fish. In the absence of further accounts it seems likely she was taught to shoot in the woodland around her home and to fish in Shawnigan Lake, which is located on the south of Vancouver Island and derives its name from the Hun'qumi'num language, which calls the lake *Shaanii'us*. Fish abundant in the lake include rainbow trout, cut-throat trout, kokanee salmon and smallmouth bass. Nowadays most fishing in Shawnigan Lake, as in most lakes in Canada and the United States, is carried out with lures. This was also the case in Frankie's day, though the lures she used would most likely have been made from wood instead of plastic. Fishing is usually from a boat out in the lake, and the bass caught there are large and fight well. It's not difficult to imagine Frankie tussling successfully with a good-sized bass of 3 or 4 pounds and taking it home to her mother for the family dinner.

Frankie enjoyed going to summer camp. Very little is known in any detail of her life in any of the camps she attended, but she reports later in her life that, when she was 12 years old, she had a summer camp friend called Bunty Bailey [sic], subsequently Mrs Janet B. Hardy.

In fact, Janet's maiden name was spelled 'Baillie'. Janet Baillie was born in Duncan, British Columbia, Canada, and grew up in Victoria, British Columbia. Her father, a doctor, once told her, 'No daughter of mine is ever going to be a physician'. Like Frankie, Janet had her own sense of her worth and chose the career she wanted: in medicine. After graduating from the University of British Columbia, she went to medical school at McGill University in Montreal, graduating in 1941 with a specialty in pediatrics. Janet came to Johns Hopkins a year later and established the first neonatal ward at its hospital. Dr Hardy spent six years as director of the Baltimore Health Department's Bureau of Child Hygiene before returning to Johns Hopkins in 1957 to direct the Collaborative Perinatal Project.

Janet subsequently established the Johns Hopkins Adolescent Pregnancy and Parenting Programs in the mid 1970s. This offered education, counseling, and access to birth control to girls at a Baltimore high school and junior high, and documented a 30-per cent drop in rates of pregnancy. At schools without the program, pregnancies reportedly increased by 58 per cent.

Janet became a Johns Hopkins University pediatrics professor. She officially retired in 1981 but continued to publish research papers well into her eighties. Like her even more illustrious childhood friend Frankie, Janet enjoyed a long life. She passed away on 23 October 2008.

Janet's brother, James Baillie, was a Canadian Second World War hero, who predeceased her by a few months, passing away on 10 August 2008.

'A keen and willing pupil with a rebellious and sometimes naughty streak' – our heroine was the savior of a large portion of mankind, but at school she could be mischievous. Four of Frankie's school reports from St George's, her boarding school in Victoria, have survived.

The first report, for the half-year ending 16 December 1927, reports on the behavior of Frances Kathleen Oldham, aged 13 and 5/12, which sounds like a Harry Potter-ish kind of age, but was at the time a routine way of indicating a child's age on a school report in Canada. Her form was the Fifth High School preliminary form. There were nineteen children in the class, and the average age was 14 years and 2 months.

When it comes to scripture, Frances is described as 'Always interested, thoughtful'. In maths she gets 'Excellent' for geometry, 'Very good' for algebra, and 'Very good indeed' for arithmetic. In English literature she only gets 'Good', and for English composition she gets 'Good on the whole'. As for history, she is depicted as 'Good, but a more accurate knowledge needed'. In French she is 'Good. Frankie works well'. In Latin she is 'Excellent' – which might help to explain why she was so au fait and adept with Latin drug names later in her career.

For drawing and brush work she only gets 'Fair'. In physical culture she is 'Very fair, Frankie has done better work this term'. As for the piano, her teacher comments, 'Would be quite good if she could only be induced to do regular patient work', which presumably means regular practice. Her overall position in the class is first – she is top of the class, with an average of 82 per cent. However, her overall conduct was not regarded by the head teacher as exemplary. As the head teacher comments:

An earnest and interested worker. Conduct under supervision excellent, but in dormitory Frankie's conduct leaves much to be desired. I should like to feel that Frankie could be relied upon to keep the few rules of the school when I am not there.

Her record of order marks at times is disgraceful for a high school girl.

Evidently when unsupervised, Frankie's high spirits could often get the better of her. Her excellent performance in academics clearly didn't transfer across to behaviour; 'order marks' are a minor punishment for misbehaving in some schools. Well, later in life, she was to achieve great things for mankind by being disobedient to an unscrupulous pharmaceutical company that wanted to walk all over her, so perhaps this report shows some indication of an early presence of a useful characteristic.

The next school report is from St Margaret's School for the term ending 28 June 1929, for the pupil described as 'Frankie Oldham', which suggests that by now Frankie was the name by which she was better known. Her position in class was second with 74 per cent. For history she gets a 'Very good', for literature now she gets 'Shows keen appreciation', for composition – apparently improved – she gets 'Very good and attentive to corrections'. For arithmetic she gets 'Fair work', but with a caveat: 'I do not like Frankie's attitude at class'. In geometry she receives 'Good work done' and in French 'Good, works well'. Her Latin is again 'Excellent', and in chemistry she is 'Good'. Her music teacher remarks that 'During last half term Frankie has proven that she *can* work. I hope this may continue'. Gymnastics was perhaps not her strong point: her gymnastics teacher comments, 'Frankie could do better work'. The form teacher at St Margaret's School now writes, 'Frankie must try to be courteous and respectful to her elders. Otherwise conduct and work are very good'. The head teacher comments: 'Frankie has improved greatly in manner and appearance during this year. She must endeavour to correct her awkward gait – a great detriment to her [illegible]'.

That final word is not legible but appears to start with the letters 'woman', although only the first three letters are definitely readable. Perhaps the word was 'womanliness'.

The third school report that has survived is also from St Margaret's School and this time for the term ending 11 April 1930. Her position in the class was second with 80 per cent. In scripture she is 'Thoughtful and interested', and for history, literature, and composition she is given an amalgamated report that states, 'Frankie sometimes attains a very high standard in these subjects, but all her work is marred by carelessness and poor spelling'. In algebra and geometry she gets 'Very good' and 'Very good indeed' respectively. In Latin authors she gets 'Does thorough and thoughtful work'. The overall verdict on Frankie for this year of school is, 'Frankie has done some very good work and results are excellent in spite of much absence'.

It's not known what the causes of the absence were, possibly bouts of ill health. The headmistress also comments, 'Frankie must realize that added responsibilities and privileges need careful consideration'. That was certainly a lesson which she learned well in later life.

The fourth and final extant report on Frankie's school life is for the term ending 19 December 1930. This time Frankie's position in the class was again first, and the average age of the class was 16 years and 1 month. Her overall performance in literature was described as 'Good, but Frankie's work would improve with a greater degree of carefulness'. For English composition she is described as 'Usually good. Examination disappointing'. In trigonometry the comment is, 'Frankie is too easily discouraged', but her results for algebra, geometry, and French were all pretty good, with her algebra teacher describing her as working 'steadily'. In chemistry the teacher remarks, 'Frankie must not be discouraged when she fails to understand some work. She is apt to magnify her own difficulties but has done a good term's work'. In music the comment is, 'Has improved', and in gymnastics the remark is, 'Deportment exceedingly poor. More physical work needed. Hockey improving'. The word 'deportment', which is now fairly obsolete in the English language on both sides of the Atlantic, meant one's general manner and way of holding oneself. The headmistress comments overall:

> Frankie is making good progress in her work. She must not worry and become too easily discouraged. As a prefect, she is most helpful. Her influence is good, and she cares for the interests of the school.

We're not suggesting that these school reports necessarily provide profound insight into Frankie's subsequent development into an adult of extraordinary importance. But they do paint a picture of an intellectually gifted young woman, who was by no means always inclined to be obedient. While this is hardly a rare characteristic of young people, it may have some significance when one considers her later life and her insistence on getting to the truth of the situation rather than kow-towing to the executives of the William S. Merrell Company.

Frankie continues her own life story:

> I graduated from high school at the age of fifteen. This might seem young, but there were two things to explain it: one was this good beginning I'd had, but the other was that we only had three years of high school in those days, so you did eleven years to get through a little earlier. I think the year after I graduated, high school became four years. My family thought I was a little young to go to college, and so the school was somehow talked into putting on 'Senior Matriculation'. In those days you could do first-year college in high school, and it was called 'Senior Matric'. I do not think that is a possibility now.

Again, we see Frankie's instinctive intellectual ambition and desire to get ahead. In her words, there is also the sense that she doesn't think being a woman places her under any handicap in where she wants to go in her career. As she also recalls in her memoir: 'I knew I wanted to go on to university, but I had not much idea what it involved'.

Recalling her two aunts, the doctor and the lawyer:

> In those days, of course, they did not practice very much, but they felt that their lives were greatly enriched by their extra education. My aunt who was a doctor took her training and then married a doctor, but she did do some laboratory work.

This short passage, and Frankie's 'of course' is extremely revealing in terms of what it says about women's intellectual careers in those days.

It was often the case that a woman might educate herself to be able to practice a particular profession but then not pursue the profession as she was going to get married and have children anyway.

Frankie adds:

> I was very surprised when I looked back at my high school scores to see that I'd gone honors in all things: composition, Latin authors, Latin composition, French translation, and French grammar – nothing about science.

One yearns to learn more about her love of Latin authors and Latin composition, and perhaps to see one of her Latin compositions, but as far as we're aware there is no record of any of those.

Frankie recalls:

> I knew I wanted to go into science, but not in chemistry; I thought it would be biology. I had no idea what biology was about, or where I could go for help. We did not have college counselors at the school at that time. Universities did not go around 'drumming up' students, and few of the girls in those days went on to college. I do not say none did. Some of them went for a year or two, admittedly for the social life. Other popular careers at that time were nursing and business college. Some girls did go on, but not enough to give me the idea to do so.

Again, we see the reference to young women studying to develop their intellect without any view to a practical application of this. That clearly was not how Frankie saw things. It's interesting that even here she sets down an inherent interest in biology rather than in chemistry. It may seem to a non-scientist that all these branches of science are equally arcane but, when all is said and done, chemistry is clearly a different kettle of fish (indeed, almost literally that) compared with biology, which is a study of life in all its complexities.

Frankie herself was intensely enthusiastic about studying biology. As she recalls, she was 'stuck another year in school with only chemistry for science', which she clearly regarded as a significant deprivation. But then things changed:

> I had a very lucky meeting in the summer, just before I was due to go back to school, with a young biology teacher, Dr Anthony Kingscote. At that time he must have been in Guelph (the Ontario College of Agriculture) returning for a holiday. He was already starting his career as a parasitologist.

According to Frankie, Dr Kingscote heard of her interest in biology and 'gave me a most marvelous overview of the field during a picnic'. If Dr Kingscote had any interest in Frankie beyond that of a willing pupil, there is no evidence. Her enthusiasm for her times with Dr Kingscote are quite clear from her memoir, written much later in her life:

> We went along the beach finding all these orders of animals and so on. Then he said there was one thing I had to do: I had to take biology in my first year of college so I could take zoology in my second, and then in my third and fourth years I could specialize and have a really good degree when I was through.

This may seem like an exciting opportunity presented to a young woman who is making crucial decisions about her future intellectual life, but Frankie recalls that in fact Kingscote's advice:

> threw me into despondency, because I was obliged to go back to school, and biology certainly would not be taught there. But it was arranged that I would go to Victoria College, drop Latin, and take biology. That was great. The wonderful teacher there, Jeff Cunningham, really stimulated me, and, if I'd gone to the University of Victoria or to the University of British Columbia, I'm sure that I would have been a marine biologist.

So vivid are Frankie's memories of those days that she even recalls what she wore.

There was one little hitch; I had to wear a school uniform, and I must have looked awfully funny in my navy blue tunic, white shirt, and long black stockings amongst all the co-eds at Victoria College dressed up to the nines. That was not the day of blue jeans in college – students dressed up. Here I was week after week in this same attire, but it was worth it and I enjoyed it.

Six

HEADING TOWARD
A VOCATION

In her second year at Victoria College, Frankie studied zoology, the specialized form of biology that focuses on the animal kingdom, including the structure, embryology, evolution, classification, habits, and distribution of all animals, both living and extinct, and how they interact with their ecosystems.

For her last two years of college, Frankie went to McGill University in Montreal, where she took specialized courses with professors who were more widely known than Jeff Cunningham at Victoria College but, as Frankie puts it: 'not to my mind nearly as stimulating'.

Frankie wondered what her particular focus should be for her senior year. She recalls that the fiancé of one of the other female students was studying medicine, and he suggested to Frankie that she try a little human biology, and take some courses with medical students.

Frankie hadn't thought of this, but it seemed like a good idea, so she signed up for biochemistry. The course included some endocrinology: the study of hormones and disorders of the endocrine system such as diabetes and hypothyroidism.

Endocrinologists typically study metabolism, growth and development, tissue function, sleep, digestion, respiration, excretion, mood, stress, lactation, movement, reproduction, and sensory perception caused by hormones. Frankie also applied herself to physiology and pharmacology.

Clearly, in view of her subsequent career, her study of pharmacology was momentous. But at the time, as Frankie recalls, her study of pharmacology was, at least for her:

> an afterthought, because I already had more credits than I needed for graduating. Somebody said, 'It is a very interesting course. You really ought to take it'. I said, 'Fine', and I signed up for it.

As she explains:

> Pharmacology ... is the study of the way chemicals act on the body. That is a general definition, and more specifically one thinks of it as the way drugs act on the body – substances that are used to cure, treat, or prevent disease.

In 1934 Frankie graduated with a bachelor of science degree. At that point, like any other graduate, she faced the challenge of wondering what to do next. She was twenty years old, and by anyone's standards in 1934, she was a highly educated woman with the world at her feet. Or at least she would have been, if the world had not been in the depths of economic depression. Frankie would have liked to have been hired by a laboratory, but as she recalls:

> There were absolutely no jobs, and the few openings there were, were almost invariably filled by men. I do not think that this was due to any particular prejudice against women. The general explanation was that men would be the supporters of the family and therefore they should have jobs first. I do not think there was a particular grievance at that time that women were overlooked, and certainly there were many men graduates that had no job to go to. This

situation led me to realize that my choices were either to do graduate studies or to join the breadline. Those were about the only alternatives in those days, and I decided that graduate work would be more interesting.

Recording her decision to embark on graduate studies, Frankie says in her memoir:

A person might wonder why I did not decide that in the first place. Well, I was a little awed. I thought one had to be really bright and brainy to be a graduate student, and, of course, that is not the case if one is interested in one's subject.

There was also a more pragmatic point:

In those days, since there was no work to get, there was no reason to hurry to get through graduate school. Graduate students stayed on and on at a low salary, working very hard at teaching and not getting all the research done that they might. Finally, I thought it was probably a good idea to go to graduate school and get a master's degree.

A memo from Frankie to Dr John Swann, dated 14 March 1996, provides insight into her studies in embryology.

I became acquainted with Dr Hartman in 1938–39 when I spent a month at the Carnegie Institute of Embryology in Baltimore studying an eight-millimeter cetacean embryo. It was the pituitary gland area that I was interested in. It was a very interesting month, and I made a plaster-of-Paris model, but unfortunately, never wrote up my findings. I did, however, publish an article on the embryology of armadillos' pituitary.

I recently [saw] a photo showing a gross specimen of an eight-millimeter porpoise and a photomicrograph of a section of the pituitary area. This was in some old photographs and negatives from Dr Geiling's collection, I believe.

Frankie found endocrinology particularly fascinating. As she explains:

> Endocrine glands pour out their secretions – or hormones – into the bloodstream, and then these act at a site distant from the gland itself. The biochemistry department at McGill was working on the pituitary gland, and until about four or five years earlier, the only thing that people thought the pituitary gland did was to influence growth. Tumors would produce very tall people, absent the gland gives dwarves. Then, in the very early 1930s, it was discovered that all sorts of exciting things were coming out of the pituitary, all sorts of hormones that stimulated other glands: the thyrotropic hormone stimulates the thyroid, the gonadotropic hormone stimulates the gonads, and so on. So the pituitary gland got the name of the master gland or, more picturesquely, the conductor of the endocrine orchestra.

This artistic way of thinking about medicine and her profession was very typical of Frankie all her adult life: she wasn't just highly skilled at a technical level in her field of expertise, she was also good at communicating aspects of it to other people.

Frankie believed that it wasn't only important to know the technical aspects of one's profession but also to be able to distill them into clear and coherent points for the layman and those in other specialties.

Unfortunately, when she went to the biochemistry department at McGill she learned there were no places available in endocrinology. As she recalls:

> I was obviously very disappointed, and the professor, taking pity on me, said, 'Why don't you go upstairs to the pharmacology department? Dr Raymond Stehle is working on the posterior lobe of the pituitary, and he does not like graduate students very much, but he might take you'.

Despite this definitely inauspicious introduction, Frankie, not someone to avoid confronting a challenge, went to the pharmacology department and spoke to Stehle. His reply, as Frankie recalls, was:

Fine, then you can be my graduate student for a year. I am not very good with graduate students, for I don't enjoy them very much, but I will be very happy to give you all the help I can.

Evidently she had charmed him with her enthusiasm and determined and energetic manner. Frankie relates:

At that time the posterior lobe was a very drab sort of affair, but the posterior and anterior are so close together in humans and other animals that you cannot exactly separate them. The posterior pituitary is actually connected to the brain by a little stalk, and if one looks at it under the microscope, it looks just like brain tissue. If injections of that are made, there are some very quick, short-term effects. A rise in blood pressure, for example, is one effect, as is stimulation of the uterus. Another effect is to cause a let-down in dairy cows so they give their milk more readily, important [for] a dairy country like Canada.

We don't imagine that anyone has ever before spoken so interestingly about a lobe of a particular gland, let alone made the ready segue to the dairy industry of Canada. Generally, there is something very Canadian about the way that Frankie, throughout her life, keeps herself rooted in everyday economic matters, especially relating to her homeland, even after she begins to work in the United States. There is also a distinct lack of pretension about how she discusses her career, partly due to her own apparent insistence on keeping her feet on the ground intellectually but also because of her generous and warm-spirited approach to life in general.

Frankie continues:

This lobe did not have the glamor in those days of the anterior pituitary so there was no one else working with Dr Stehle. But I had anticipated the interest, and in the last ten or twenty years the posterior pituitary has come into its own. At that time it was not thought that the brain could give rise to secretions, but now it is an accepted fact that it does. We now know the posterior lobe secretions actually control the anterior lobe; I do not know whether it should be called the super-conductor or what. That was not so in my day; it was not a particularly prominent organ to work on.

Frankie's investigations of the anterior pituitary lobe were thorough, as all her work was. She recalls that when she studied the operation of the anterior lobe, she encountered two fundamental problems:

> One was whether all these different effects were caused just by one chemical or by several forms. That is what Dr Stehle and colleagues were working on. The other problem was where these chemicals came from. Did they indeed come from the brain, or did they come from the anterior lobe and just drift into the posterior lobe? That is the research I came to later. With Dr Stehle, I studied the effects of the posterior pituitary on the water balance of frogs, and that was a topic of my thesis. For a year I sat surrounded by frogs in little cages set in water. I would lift them up, dry them, weigh them, inject them, put them back in the water, and then weigh them at fifteen to twenty minute intervals for four hours. I would get the most beautiful curves on graphs; I was able to find out which part of the extract causes particular effects.

Frankie received her master's degree in a year, but then was faced with the same problem she had confronted before: there was no job for her anywhere. However, Dr Stehle had a grant, and he told Frankie he was happy to pay her 50 dollars a month to be his research assistant while she looked for another position. He told Frankie that if she received an offer for another position, she should take it.

Frankie, though, stuck with him. As she recalls:

> Believe it or not, fifty dollars a month was a sum that one could live on, not lavishly, but adequately. So, I lived on that and continued working for Dr Stehle on the posterior pituitary.

Frankie lived on this modest stipend. Then, in February 1936, Dr Stehle told her he had learned that a new pharmacology department was opening at the University of Chicago. The professor who had been hired there as chairman, a Dr Eugene Geiling from John Hopkins University, had also been doing work on the posterior pituitary gland. Stehle thought Geiling might be interested in Frankie because of her work in this field. Stehle advised Frankie to write to Geiling and ask him if he wanted a research assistant; she also could perhaps explain to Geiling that she was interested in getting a PhD or a fellowship.

> So I did. Postage was three cents in those days. Not much was lost, and my hopes were not very high, but to my great surprise I got back a letter Air Mail, Special Delivery, on February 15 (I remember the date). It said: 'If you can be in Chicago by March first, you may have the research assistantship for four months and then a scholarship to see you through a PhD. Please wire immediate decision'.

The year was 1936. Frankie clearly had a vivid memory of this letter, sent by special delivery, and it turned out to play a major role in her career development.

Yet the question was, had Dr Geiling offered the opportunity to a woman or a man? Frankie herself raised that matter for the following reason:

> There was just one thing that bothered me a little about that letter. It started out, 'Dear Mr. Oldham', and here my conscience tweaked me a bit. I knew that men were the preferred commodity in those days. Should I write and explain that Frances with an *e* is female and with an *I* is male?

Evidently flummoxed by this dilemma, she asked Stehle for his advice. As she recalls, he said:

> Don't be ridiculous. Accept the job, sign your name, put Miss in brackets afterwards, and go!

A pragmatic plan indeed and as Frankie remembers:

> That is what I did, and, to this day, I do not know if my name had been
> Elizabeth or Mary Jane, whether I would have gotten that first big step up.
> My professor at Chicago to his dying day would never admit one way or the
> other.

Does Frankie's remark mean that, on at least one occasion, she asked
Dr Geiling about whether he initially thought he was corresponding
with a man? It seems that very likely she did, but either way, he never
told her the truth. Perhaps he was embarrassed that he had indeed assumed she was a man until he got her reply. This possibility seems all the
more likely, given Frankie's comments about the man who played such
an important role in developing her career:

> Dr Geiling was very conservative and old-fashioned. He really did not hold
> too much with women as scientists. But he was very fair, and a number of
> women graduated in his departments while he was professor at Chicago. I was
> his first PhD student. I went to the University of Chicago in March of 1936.

Frankie was fascinated from the outset by her work with Geiling.

> The work that Dr Geiling was doing concerned whether these posterior
> pituitary hormones came from the posterior lobe or the anterior lobe ...
> He did not think it unreasonable to think that nerve tissue could make
> hormones; other people thought otherwise. He thought one way to prove
> his point would be to find an animal in which the anterior [pituitary] lobe
> and the posterior lobe were completely separated so that it could not be said
> that the activities would diffuse from one to the other.

Frankie adds, now giving her memoir a decidedly zoological aspect:

By the time I worked for him, he had found this to be the case in the armadillo, the whale, the porpoise, and in birds and seals. My work was with the
armadillo, and that is what I did my PhD on: the anatomy and the pharmacology of the posterior pituitary gland of the nine-banded armadillo.

Frankie remarked in her memoir that the armadillo is 'not one of your
common laboratory animals'. The armadillo had often aroused the
interest of researchers because, 'for some reason or another they always
had genetically identical quadruplets, so the geneticists were interested'.

Frankie completed her PhD on the subject of the adult armadillo. She
received her degree in 1938, which she followed with a year's post-graduate
study on why these two lobes were separate, which meant studying the
embryos of armadillos. As she explains:

Armadillos have a very weird cycle, and there is no way they can be bred in
the laboratory. We had to get our supplies from Texas at that time. Possibly
that is still done. There was an armadillo farm in Texas, very close to the
Lyndon Baines Johnson ranch. They used to ship the armadillos up to us.
On one occasion when I wanted to study embryo armadillos, I had to go
down to the armadillo farm in Texas to hunt and catch a few to get my
embryonic armadillos.

It's clear that some aspects of Frankie's work involved killing armadillos
in order to pursue her research. She adopts a pragmatic attitude toward
this. While vivisection is regarded as less acceptable today than it was
in Frankie's time, it is still a necessity to pursue various types of medical
research.

At one point in her research Frankie was also involved in getting
samples of organs from whales. She pointed out that the one whale organ
it was not possible to bring back to the laboratory was the heart, as it
would weigh between 200 and 300 pounds. She recalls that during two
summers at this time she got to go to a whaling station at Rose Harbor.

The whales were caught by ninety-foot boats. I think they had a crew of about eleven or thirteen, and the harpoon gun was at the bow. Now the great adventure each year, for the scientists going out there, was to be able to go out in a whale boat. The first year I was there, I heard every excuse under the sun, 'It was a bad day, this, that, and the other', and I could not go in the boat. The second year I was able to go, and I think, in part, it was because the son of the manager was spending his summers working on that boat, and he used to keep an eye on me.

Frankie recalls this expedition with great vividness:

It was a lovely day, early in the morning, and he very kindly took me up in the barrel [a literal barrel high up in the boat from which it was possible to have a good lookout] with him, and we spotted a sperm whale. The different kinds of whales could be distinguished by the spout. I cannot remember the differences now, but I know that is how you tell. We directed the helmsmen, the harpooner and everything, and we got the whale. Now, I did not realize how lucky I was, because I learned the reason I had not been able to go before was that whalers are very superstitious, and one of the superstitions was that having a woman on board a whaling vessel brings bad luck. This was important to the crew because a certain amount of their pay was based on the number and type of whale that was caught. At least I think I broke that jinx.

Frankie broke another precedent too as she recalls:

I did score another mark for women in that I was the only scientist taken out on these whaling expeditions who was not violently seasick.

Frankie's interest in whales was complemented by her work with the ling cod, a hefty fish that is also known as the buffalo cod – appropriately in view of the fact that it can weigh as much as 130 pounds. But as Frankie explains, she became interested in the ling cod for other reasons:

It was known that the pancreas [of a ling cod] has a rather unusually high level of zinc in it compared to other parts of its body. It was not a dramatically high amount, and it was quite difficult to measure because it was so slight. But it was distinctly higher than in certain other parts of the body. The pancreas, like the pituitary, really is a two-part organ. There is the main body, the main pancreas, that secretes the digestion enzymes and pours them into the intestine, and then scattered amongst these are little islets of tissue that were long thought to be where insulin came from. But this was pretty hard to prove because when the pancreas was ground up, the enzymes ate up the insulin, so there was nothing to be measured. That was a problem.

Frankie also recalls:

The question of where the insulin came from was solved very neatly by Dr Macleod, who was at the University of Toronto and later, of course, got the Nobel Prize for his work on insulin.

Most people associate Dr Frederick Banting with successfully isolating insulin, which pioneered an effective treatment for diabetes. Before insulin was discovered and made available, the disease was almost invariably fatal. In fact, the 1923 Nobel Prize in Physiology or Medicine was awarded jointly to Dr Macleod and Dr Banting. Macleod's award was controversial at the time; according to Banting's version of events, Macleod's role in the discovery was negligible, and it was only decades later that an independent review attributed to him a greater role. Thus Frankie's identification of Macleod as a crucial pioneer in insulin research was, in many respects, against the general prevailing trend of thought at the time. In her memoir, Frankie identifies Dr Macleod's research with his work with the ling cod and other fish:

He was aware that in certain fish the islet tissue was an entirely separate organ (a little sort of pea-like body) quite apart from the rest of the pancreas. He extracted these little islets, and sure enough he was able to get the blood-sugar-lowering effect of insulin. That clinched the question of whether the insulin came from these tissues.

Frankie had managed to forge a successful, if not yet especially distinguished, career in medical research. In her memoir she now touches on the professional area that would eventually be such a major part of her life: the investigation and regulation of new drugs.

Seven

TRAGEDY AND FOCUS

Frankie's first introduction to problems with new drugs came about in September 1937, not long after she arrived at the University of Chicago. We have already looked at this particular medical catastrophe, but it's interesting to view it from Frankie's own perspective. As she says:

> Sulfanilamide had been introduced about 1933 in Germany. It was the wonder drug; it completely changed the face of medicine. Here was something that would actually attack some infectious germs and save many lives. People who previously would have died of pneumonia, or streptococcus or staphylococcus infections and so on, were saved by this new drug. Its use spread very rapidly all over the world – so fast that no basic scientific work had really been done on this drug. But it had drawbacks, the patient had to take a large dose, the pills were pretty unpalatable and disagreeable to take, it caused gastrointestinal upset, and so on.

Frankie then gets to the hub of the tragedy:

One manufacturer had a great idea. It was decided to put up a liquid solution, which would be easy to take and which would be particularly agreeable to children. Now the drug is not soluble in either alcohol or water, which most drug solutions are made up in, so the company officials had their chemists go along the shelves and find a solvent that would dissolve the sulfanilamide. I guess the first thing the manufacturer found that was successful was diethylene glycol, which is antifreeze. This was not tested on animals and the liquid form of the drug was just put right on the market ... Then the reports came in of fatalities. One doctor in a small town had five patients die in a short space of time. They were all taking this drug. People knew so little about sulfanilamide, they were not sure whether it was the sulfanilamide or the solvent that was causing the deaths.

As we've seen, it was diethylene glycol that was responsible for the problem. It shut down the kidneys permanently. This was discovered by Dr Geiling and Frankie working together. As she explains:

Dr Geiling had worked with the Food and Drug Administration previously, when he had been in Baltimore, helping them in other cases, some of which he used to describe in his toxicology classes. So the FDA called him up and said, 'Help us out!'

At the time, the FDA did not have its own resources that would let it evaluate what was responsible for the deaths. Geiling immediately set up animal studies for acute and chronic toxicity. Frankie was responsible for documenting the effects that the solution had on the rats. She found that rats that were given diethylene glycol or the solution that had been marketed by Massengill gradually stopped producing urine because their kidneys stopped functioning. The research which Geiling undertook and to which Frankie contributed gave Frankie a good understanding of the principle that animal tests can be highly effective in predicting likely toxicity of new drugs (or of any drugs).

The precise reason for the toxic effects of diethylene glycol are still not completely understood even today. Toxicology is an extremely complex science, and it is almost always much easier to state that a chemical *is* toxic than to understand conclusively *why* it is. In the case of diethylene glycol, the chemical interferes with a variety of bodily processes, in particular kidney and liver function.

Frankie gained her PhD in 1938, after which she carried out some post-graduate work, but she still wanted to find a real job. She thought of going back to Canada, but that came to nothing. She began to wonder whether she would have had more opportunities in her profession if she were a man; jobs for women were very hard to come by. But then, the Second World War arrived, and that changed the whole situation, not just for scientists, but for everyone; 'No longer could a person hope to get by or get an interesting job without a good educational background'. Suddenly Frankie's determination to become well-educated began to make real sense.

She relates what happened next:

> Quite suddenly a group working under Dr Geiling at the University of Chicago got involved in a big project to find new anti-malarial drugs ... . Obviously malaria was a serious problem in wartime, and of course World War II had broken out by that time. But then with the fall of the Dutch East Indies, 90 per cent of the world's supply of quinine, at least for the Allies, disappeared. There was one other drug available, a German drug called Atabrine, but it was considered pretty toxic, and people did not like to take it. So there had to be a crash program to get some other treatment for malaria.

There were efforts to synthesize an American version of Atabrine that would not be toxic. These efforts were reasonably successful, but efforts to synthesize quinine had failed: it was a very tedious process with a low yield. Frankie remarks that such a process has never, as far as she knows, become economically feasible.

Frankie and her team worked hard to try to develop new drugs to combat malaria. In any event, Frankie had at last managed to gain some regular employment and was working on this project from 1941 to 1945, while the Second World War raged. During this period, Frankie met a colleague, a doctor called Fremont Ellis Kelsey.

Eight

MARRIAGE AND
MOTHERHOOD

Dr Fremont Ellis Kelsey was an instructor at the University of Chicago and held a PhD in biochemistry from the University of Rochester.

Frankie and Ellis's younger daughter Christine Kelsey says:

> I don't know much about their courtship. They worked together on many projects in the lab, including the war research on malaria, they had many mutual friends, and they went to plays in Chicago.

As far as we are aware, there is nothing else known for sure about their courtship, but it's reasonable to suppose that it was founded on a deep intellectual and professional congeniality. What is certain is that Frankie and Ellis were married on Monday, 6 December 1943, at the Church of the Redeemer on 1420 East 56th Street, Chicago. The priest who married them was the Reverend Edward S. White and the witnesses were Julius M. Coon and Monica Oldham.

Monica, Frankie's younger sister, was born in May 1923, and died in Victoria in July 2017. Monica grew up in Cobble Hill, on a small hobby farm, during the economic depression of the 1930s. After completing high school at Queen Margaret's, she attended the Banff School of Fine Arts. In her early twenties she trained as an occupational therapist. A lady with an unfailingly adventurous and inquisitive personality, as a young woman, she traveled throughout Europe and Australia and worked on a ranch in Montana. Like Frankie, Monica was blessed with a strong social conscience and an awareness of what human greed can lead to. One obituary of Monica said:

> Monica never cowed to social convention, she lived with the integrity of her philosophy 'take only what you need, no more and NEVER waste'. Through-out her life in her professional work and as an activist, she was concerned with the long-term impacts of human greed on the environment and hu-man communities. Monica never shied from an opportunity to debate and educate. Compassionate and loyal, she understood the deeper truths in life.

Meanwhile, in Europe, the war raged on. On 6 December 1943, that same day Frankie and Ellis got married, the first Jews were shipped out of Italy on a train taking innocent prisoners from Milan to Verona and then to Auschwitz. At the Jaworzno concentration camp in Poland, between nineteen and twenty-nine inmates were hanged in front of other inmates for participating in building an escape tunnel.

When the nightmare of the Second World War finally ended and there was less of a sense of emergency in Frankie's department, a problem arose: two members of the same family in those days could not be employed in the same department at the university.

As a result, Frankie and Ellis decided that the best solution would be for one of them to go to medical school and get an MD. They decided that Frankie would be the one to do this because she had already studied two years of medicine while getting her PhD. She also wanted to maximize her credentials and qualifications in hopes of obtaining another job, given that she couldn't continue working at the University of Chicago. In 1946 Frankie went to medical school at the University of Chicago while Ellis continued his teaching and research in the department of pharmacology.

As Frankie recalls:

Medical school was not bad, because this was the first year after the war, [and] students were much older. On the average, they were aged twenty-seven, instead of twenty-one or twenty. They were much more mature, and less likely to rag the women. Then, because of the scarcity of men, there was a higher per centage of women in the class. There were seven of us for seventy places (ten per cent), and earlier, only one or two per year would get in. So, medical school was not bad as far as I was concerned, particularly, as we had some very fine women professors on the staff, who had the respect of their male counterparts. Furthermore, the university medical school at Chicago was oriented more for teaching and research than for private practice. Again, the atmosphere was not as competitive.

Susan Elizabeth Kelsey, the Kelseys' first child, was born at Chicago Lying-In Hospital (attached to the University of Chicago) in 1947. The Kelseys' second child, Christine Ann Kelsey, was born in 1949, also at Chicago Lying-In Hospital. Frankie was fortunate to be able to get a considerable amount of time off for maternity purposes. As she explains:

Chicago was on a quarter system, so it was possible to have three quarters on and one quarter off. You could choose your quarters, more or less; it was very flexible, so it was ideal timing.

But as Christine Kelsey told us, this time off for maternity leave was unpaid.

In the light of the most significant and important professional project of her life, one particular comment she makes in her memoir has considerable resonance:

I was very cautious about using drugs during my own pregnancies. I do not smoke, so that never came up, and in those times I do not think we could afford to do much drinking.

Clearly, Frankie had no doubt whatsoever that substances such as prescription drugs and alcohol could cross the placental barrier. As she was writing of a time here – thirteen and eleven years before she was asked to evaluate the thalidomide new drug application (NDA) – this again shows that doctors were aware of drugs crossing the placental barrier. All the protests by those involved with manufacturing and developing thalidomide are at best founded on shaky ground and at worst indicate a complete indifference on the part of greedy executives to what thalidomide might do to unborn children.

Frankie did not plan to practice medicine. Instead she wanted to work in a medically related field. Even before she gained her medical degree, Frankie had applied for a job at the American Medical Association as an editorial associate at *The Journal of the American Medical Association*. The new editor there was a Canadian, Dr Austin Smith, who had trained in Toronto and was a pharmacologist. Frankie knew him because he had an appointment at the University of Chicago in the Pharmacology Department. As she recalls:

He would give several lectures a year. Dr Geiling was always anxious to get outside persons to have at least part-time faculty appointments so there would be intermixing to broaden the scope of the department and give us these contacts.

Austin Smith felt there should be more articles in the *Journal* about new drugs, but he also felt that the caliber of writing for many of the articles submitted was not very good. Frankie's job was to pick out good papers from those submitted and to help the office polish them up. She recalled, rather ruefully:

Not all the science was very good either, and I do not know if I was very successful in that line, but my main job was to try and pick good papers, and I hope I did that.

[...] We all agreed that many of the submissions were poor, and we also observed that no matter whether we turned them down or not, they inevitably got published in some other journal, because the journals circulated amongst us. We would see these articles and realize that we had reviewed them and recommended they not be accepted. Certain names would keep recurring, both in articles and things like letters and so forth. We kept a sort of informal list. We would jot down, 'Oh it's Dr So-and-So again' or 'So-and-So...' Eight years later, when I came to the Food and Drug Administration (FDA), I saw many familiar names as contributors of clinical studies to the NDAs. I have to be honest and admit that there were some articles I turned down then but now would have accepted, but I think that is true of all editors. I am glad to say that those articles too got published.

Frankie was at the AMA for two years (from 1952–1954), and then Ellis received an offer to be head of the Pharmacology Department at the University of South Dakota Medical School in Vermillion, South Dakota.

Frankie herself was not allowed to work at the same university in Ellis's department due to the same rule in Chicago that married couples were not allowed to work in the same department. Since she did not want to practice medicine (or, as she put it, 'I was not sure if I did,') she regarded the decision to go and live in South Dakota as a significant one for the family: it meant that, initially at least, she would not have a job. Frankie debated whether to go to law school – she always said that she liked studying – or to take an internship at a medical practice. She thought it was possible that she might, after all, enjoy practicing medicine, although that was something she had never intended to do.

The Kelsey family moved to South Dakota in the summer of 1952. Early in 1953 – Frankie remembers this as being in January or February

– she started an internship at Sacred Heart Hospital, about ten miles from Vermillion at Yankton. She had decided to try an internship at the hospital and see how it went. Later in her life she recalled the internship as a 'very good experience'. When the internship came to an end, she applied for and was awarded a three-year teaching fellowship, paid for by the large drug company Lederle.

The Lederle fellowships were designed to support faculty members at universities in a way that didn't restrict the type of research they could pursue. The aim of the fellowships was to upgrade the overall quality of teaching basic sciences in medical schools. It was, as Frankie recalls,

> a very generous fellowship, and it did not cause a conflict with two people in the department being paid by the university, because I was paid by an outside firm. So, it was possible for me to spend three years doing research and teaching by virtue of my fellowship. This was from 1954 to 1957.

Frankie eventually got involved in the new field of radioisotopes and radioisotope drugs herself; there was some interest in isotopes and nuclear medicine, so she commuted to Chicago to get training in that. The commute involved an overnight train trip, and she would typically stay in Chicago for two or three days to watch and assist and then return to Vermillion.

After Frankie's Lederle fellowship ran out in 1957, she worked part-time as a volunteer medical researcher and also carried out what was known then as 'practice sitting'. As she says:

> This was somewhat like babysitting. There were many rural areas where only one doctor would be available, so when the physician wished to get away to go to a medical meeting or take a vacation, I would go and look after his practice for varying periods, say two or three days. I think the longest period I did this for was about six or eight weeks when the people in the town were looking for a replacement for a doctor in one of these areas.

We might wonder why Frankie didn't set up her own medical practice, but as she explains:

> I did this [practice sitting] rather than open my own practice, because I somehow felt that would tie me down, and the girls were still fairly young. Plus I enjoyed teaching – and did some of that too. I rather enjoyed the amount of [medical] practice I did. It offered a variety, and it was not too defining. Also, I did still have a contact at the university.

After Frankie and her family had been in Vermillion for some time, she and her husband decided they wanted to go back to big city life again. This time she got the first job offer and she recalls that she had cold feet at the idea of being the sole support of the family until Ellis got a job. Fortunately, not long after, Ellis was offered a position by the National Institutes of Health. In 1960 the family moved to Washington, D.C., where both the jobs were located.

Frankie's job offer was from the Food and Drug Administration, the federal agency that regulated the supply of food and drugs in the United States. For Frankie, it was just another job, albeit a potentially deeply interesting one. For the story of medicine and for approximately 100,000 mothers in the United States and their babies, it was, in hindsight, a job appointment of almost unimaginable importance. As the poet John Milton might have expressed it, a great angel had finally stopped standing and waiting.

Nine

A NEW RECRUIT AT THE FOOD AND DRUG ADMINISTRATION

The job offer Frankie had received came from a Dr Ralph Smith, a Canadian and a pharmacologist like Frankie. At the time he was the director of the Bureau of Medicine, the part of the FDA that included its human drugs regulatory functions. Frankie had met Dr Smith at a meeting of pharmacologists. He explained to Frankie after the meeting that the FDA was expanding and asked her whether she would like to work there as a medical officer.

> It did not seem like a bad idea, and so I mulled it over. When my husband got the job offer in Washington too, I accepted. Just to show how the job market had changed, I also got an offer from the National Institutes of Health for another job at the same time, so things were looking up.

Frankie started work at the FDA on Monday, 1 August 1960. At the time, the organization was located in a temporary building called the Wake Building, in the area of Washington where, today, the Robert F. Kennedy Memorial Stadium is located. However, at the end of August, Frankie and her colleagues were relocated into other temporary buildings on the Mall on Seventh Street, close to the Department of Health, Education, and Welfare building. These were the Second World War temporary buildings – prefabs – and as Frankie laconically remarks, 'We were lucky because some government agents were still in the First World War prefabs'.

When Frankie started work at the FDA, it was a much smaller organization than it is today, though still a considerable entity. It had about 1,100 employees in 1960. As Frankie recalls:

> My first month was spent going around and finding out what the parts of the agency did, and then I came back to our little pre-fab. Only the Bureau of Medicine was in it; other parts of the agency had bigger buildings. After my short indoctrination period, I was given my first assignments as a reviewer of new drug applications. I had been hired as a medical officer, and this meant that I would review the medical part rather than the pharmacology of new drug applications. Dr Smith, who brought me in, was looking for medical officers, not pharmacologists.

By 'medical part' Frankie means matters relating to the testing of drugs on people.

> I had the medical training as well as my pharmacological training, and there were certain advantages to being a medical officer at that time. In those days pharmacologists were not actually in the Bureau of Medicine, but in, I believe it was called, the Bureau of Science. They used to work with the Bureau of Medicine people. We would send our applications over there for them to review the animal work. So my review work was to be on the human studies from the start.

When Frankie joined the FDA, a drug firm that felt it had a drug that was ready to be marketed had to complete a new drug application: a compilation of material prepared by the drug company to basically show that the drug was safe for its proposed use or uses. As Frankie explains:

[The NDA] would consist of three parts. There would be a chemistry part which described the drug, how it was made, what different ingredients went into it, how the manufacturer would ensure purity at all steps along the way, how they would ensure that the drug would always be the same each time they made it, how stable it was – these and various other sundry aspects would come under the chemistry part. The chemists in our group reviewed that part.

Frankie also explains:

Then there would be pharmacology – the animal studies that had been done to show the drug was safe. These studies would usually be to test for acute toxicity, in which a single dose of varying amounts was given to animals – usually rats, mice, or dogs – in essence to see how little killed them rather than how much they could tolerate. What is usually done is to have a large group of animals and then determine the dose which will kill half of them. This is the LD-50. [LD stands for lethal dose.] If the dose that would kill all of them had to be found, there would always be a few very resistant ones. At the other end, if it was a dose that would kill the least number, there would always be a few sensitive ones. Instead, a fairly large group of animals was selected, and then the researcher would see at what cut-off point 50 per cent of them survived, or to say it the other way, at what point 50 per cent died. That would be the LD-50.

The third part of the procedure would be the clinical trials, which involved the drug being distributed to physicians who were supposed to be adequately trained. The physicians were then supposed to make careful observations and honestly record their findings at the trials.

By the time Frankie joined the FDA, there was a general feeling that clinical trials were often poorly performed by drug companies. Frankie goes so far as to say, 'As a newcomer I must say I was quite shocked sometimes at the caliber of the work that had gone into the application in support of safety'.

This fundamental problem, that the NDAs were often of poor quality, was not helped by the fact that working at the FDA was not seen as a high-status job by medical professionals. Frankie recalls:

> It was very difficult in those days to get people to work as medical officers in the government. The pay was very low compared to what a physician could earn elsewhere, and many physicians did not like this type of desk work. The FDA depended a lot, for example, on people who had just completed their residencies and were starting out in practice in town and would give half a day to review an application. There would be a pretty big turnover of physicians going to, say, drug firms.

This, Frankie explains, was only to be expected: the same type of skills that were utilized at the FDA were required by the drug firms, and naturally the drug firms paid considerably more than the FDA did.

Frankie's immediate supervisor at the FDA was Dr Ralph Smith himself. There was also a Dr Irwin Siegel, who was Dr Smith's deputy and had a lot to do with training new people. Frankie often went to him when she had problems, and only after then to Dr Smith. As she recalls of her workload at the FDA:

> I was not swamped with too much work at first. I cannot remember the application load at that time, but it was nothing like it is now with the investigation of drug exemptions and much larger new drug applications that the medical officers have to evaluate.

When Frankie says 'now' in this context, she means the FDA in general in subsequent decades, but especially in the 1980s and 1990s. As she explains about these more recent decades at the FDA:

> The volume of the NDAs has increased. For example, the thalidomide NDA was four volumes; now the NDAs come in 150 to 200 volumes or more.

I would describe a volume as a metropolitan phone book in size. That gives an idea of strictness. The increase in size of NDAs is certainly, in part, due to the more detail required to establish both safety and now, of course, efficacy as well.

It is fair to say that when Frankie began her new job, the FDA was not only offering poor pay and a marginally low status, but generally even had a somewhat low profile in the American medical industry itself. Certainly, Merrell clearly saw the FDA as little more than a nuisance that they needed to get past before they could achieve their commercial dreams of flooding the United States with thalidomide. Merrell came to believe, though it was soon disabused of this belief, that Frankie wouldn't be much of an obstacle, and that it wouldn't be long before thalidomide was approved for marketing and distribution in the United States.

I joined the FDA on August 1, 1960, and I think I got the thalidomide application in early September 1960. I believe it was the second one that was given to me. I was the newest person there and pretty green, so my supervisor decided: 'Well, this is a very easy one. There will be no problems with sleeping pills'.

So that is how I happened to get the application. I never got another one quite like that one. I know the other drug given to me at the same time was a rectal enema which I think had the name of 'Lavema'. It did get marketed, so I must have approved it.

Frankie's experiences with the thalidomide application were very different. She had no way of knowing this at the time, but the central drama of her life was about to start. At the heart of this drama was a simple question: were a hundred thousand American babies going to be born with grotesque deformities?

Ten

THE THALIDOMIDE NEW DRUG APPLICATION

Chemie Grünenthal licensed Merrell to distribute thalidomide in the United States and Canada in 1958, after Smith, Kline & French declined Chemie Grünenthal's offer to be the United States distributor. Smith, Kline & French's reason for declining appears to have been that its testing of thalidomide revealed no improvement in efficacy over existing drugs. Thalidomide, which was to be marketed in the United States under the trade name Kevadon, was assigned the code name MER 32 by Merrell. The company planned to begin selling thalidomide in March 1961; meeting this target would require rapid consideration and approval of its NDA by the FDA. Thalidomide had been approved for sale in Germany and England, but US law required Merrell to conduct its own studies of the safety of thalidomide.

Merrell's focus in its clinical study was principally on marketing and promotion rather than scientific inquiry. Merrell perverted the regulatory process in order to gain a head start in establishing thalidomide as a major new tranquilizer. In the words of a brochure it prepared to educate its employees about the effort, Merrell's studies, performed by private clinicians, were 'to contact Teaching Hospitals ... for the purpose of selling them Kevadon and providing them with a clinical supply'.

The thalidomide studies were conducted by Merrell's marketing department rather than its medical department. The medical department's role was limited to a veto power over the clinicians invited to participate. Merrell instructed the salespeople contacting the clinical investigators that 'the main purpose is to establish local studies whose results will be spread among hospital staff members'. Investigators could choose not to report results, an unthinkable proviso for any serious study. Placebos were only provided to investigators who requested them. The simple truth of the matter was that Merrell was far more interested in making money from thalidomide than in making sure it was safe.

Frankie's responsibility was to review the thalidomide NDA. At that time, FDA rules stipulated that such officials had sixty days after receipt of the NDA to decide whether to reject it or, if they raised no objection or missed the deadline, the drug automatically would be approved, and the company could put it on the market.

So in effect the regulatory procedure of the FDA depended on an official raising an objection. In hindsight, this was an extremely hazardous procedure. If Frankie had suddenly fallen ill or been involved in some kind of accident, the thalidomide NDA might have been approved automatically without further reference to her – and if this automatic approval had been granted, permission to market thalidomide throughout the US might not have been rescinded.

In practice, FDA officials, often quite late in the sixty-day timeframe, frequently raised the objection that the application was incomplete and detailed the deficiencies in the application. The applicant would then have to address those deficiencies before approval could take place. As Frankie recalls:

There would, of course, be a prod on the fifty-ninth day after the arrival of every application to make sure that at least some letter had been issued to the firm if there was a matter for concern. There was always the fear that through somebody being asleep at the switch the sixty days might go by and then the approval would be automatic. I understand it had happened once.

There was definitely a sense of onus on the officials of the FDA to be 'pretty specific' in saying that an application was incomplete. Reviewers had to be fair about this, and the FDA frowned on holding an application until the sixty days were almost up and then making a complaint about some aspect of it being incomplete. In the case of the thalidomide NDA, Frankie instinctively felt she wanted to delay her decision for as long as she could, until more information became available about the drug.

Still, at this early stage in her evaluation of the NDA, Frankie did not appear to have had any reason to suspect that thalidomide was anything other than the sedative Merrell claimed it to be. However, she was determined to submit the NDA to the rigorous evaluation and scrutiny that she rightly saw as the hallmark of the FDA and the professionals who worked there. Indeed, 'Scrutiny' might be an alternative title not only for this chapter, but for this entire book. As Frankie recalls: 'In general, we were supposed to do an honest and fair review'.

At the FDA, the thalidomide NDA was reviewed by three people: a chemist, a pharmacologist who was responsible for looking at the animal testing, and a medical officer, who in this case was Frankie herself. The chemist was Lee Geismar (a woman) and the pharmacologist was Jiro Oyama. As Frankie explains:

Unfortunately, in those days, we were separated. We were not much of a team, although Lee Geismar and I were in the same building, and I'm sure we would go to meetings together. In those days the medical officers actually got great support from the chemists who were the ones, in a way, who instructed us more than anyone else did in the art of drawing up these letters to the drug companies.

Frankie, Geismar and Oyama encountered problems when they initially reviewed the thalidomide NDA. Geismar's review in particular showed there were some matters she wanted to see cleared up. Frankie was especially interested in her response to the thalidomide application because Geismar had been trained in Germany and could read German.

Because thalidomide was originally made by the German firm Chemie Grünenthal, many of the documents included in thalidomide submissions were in German. Before sending it to the FDA, Merrell had been required to translate the German material into English. Geismar had been born in Stuttgart, Germany, and thus was able to refer to the original German documents. She often found that Merrell had made mistakes in the translation. It is also unclear whether *all* the documents supplied by Merrell actually had been translated into English. Frankie remarked that it was 'very handy having someone who could read foreign languages, because many of these early chemical studies were done in Germany'.

The more Frankie scrutinized the thalidomide NDA, the more unsatisfactory she found it. She was determined to ascertain beyond any reasonable doubt that it was as effective as was claimed, and that it didn't come with any downsides. After all, it wasn't as if thalidomide was purported to offer a life-saving treatment for some kind of cancer; it was simply billed as a powerful sedative. And therein lies the great irony at the core of our story.

But let's pass over that for the time being and focus on Frankie, in whose perceptive, meticulous and intellectually adventurous mind the first few uncomfortable doubts were slowly simmering.

Frankie found that the claims made in the thalidomide NDA simply seemed to be 'too glowing' and lacked support in the way of clinical backup. This was a major reason why she wanted more substantiation. As she puts it:

The claims were just not supported by the type of clinical studies that had been submitted in the application. I cannot remember what the exact number of doctors' reports in the initial submission was. I think about thirty, and many of them were more testimonials than scientific studies.

Writing about this crucial time at the FDA, Frankie emphasized that even if an NDA had satisfied the pharmacologist's criteria or the FDA's criteria on pharmacological work, the NDA would not be approved if the clinical part was still poor,. Frankie told Merrell that the FDA had queries regarding the chemical, pharmacological and clinical aspects of the application and therefore wanted the NDA to be resubmitted.

Frankie's main contact at Merrell, Dr Joseph Murray, had a background in bacteriology. He found Frankie annoying and frustrating from the outset. What was this woman doing interfering with Merrell's very reasonable plans to bring the benefit of its wonder drug to American mothers? Frankie, recalling her first contacts with Murray, says:

I think he was quite frustrated, to put it mildly, by the problems raised in the review. I suppose he had been given the responsibility of getting the [thalidomide] NDA approved as quickly as possible, and to have these road blocks thrown up must have been quite annoying.

Hardly anything is known about Dr Joseph Murray after his involvement with the thalidomide scandal; he disappears from the historical record like an evoked ghost whose purpose, having been frustrated by Frankie, vanishes into the underworld. It's important to emphasize that he is not the eminent surgeon Dr Joseph Murray who, on 23 December 1954, performed the world's first successful renal transplant between two identical twins, thus pioneering the technique for kidney transplants.

Frankie recalls:

My first dissatisfaction with the thalidomide application centered on the quality of the clinical reports, because they were more in the nature of testimonials rather than well-designed, well-executed studies. I requested Merrell, I believe, to get better clinical studies and to provide us with a little better evidence of these various and sundry claims that they had made.

In her memoir, Frankie observes that thalidomide had been marketed and 'very widely distributed in Europe' since about 1957.

Did Merrell have too great an access to her when she was evaluating the thalidomide NDA? Later in her life, Frankie said:

That is a rather hard question to answer because one has to be fair and see their interests. Many of the drug companies genuinely feel that they have a really good drug (and occasionally they do), and they have spent a lot of time getting these applications ready – lining up the people to do the work, getting the animal studies, etc. – so their hopes are riding high.

In fact, both here and elsewhere when she recalls what happened, Frankie is extremely measured in her depiction of Murray and Merrell. The company undeniably showed incompetence and dishonesty when it failed to carry out its professional and human duty to make sure that thalidomide was safe for the United States public. What Charles Dickens says in *Dombey & Son* (1848) of his character Major Bagstock might apply to Merrell too: at the heart – or perhaps 'at the stomach' is a better expression, as Merrell appeared to have had far more of the latter organ than of the former – of the slapdash approach Merrell brought to the NDA for thalidomide was the sheer desire to profit from the drug as soon as possible. Frankie is more restrained in her comments about Merrell than we might be:

With thalidomide, because it has been successfully marketed in Europe, I think one of the possible reasons why Merrell's application was so poor was that it seemed like a sort of pushover; it would have no problem at all being approved. Perhaps they had not given the application the attention it deserved, such as getting the best people as investigators, which is a standard approach in the case of an unknown drug. It is necessary in the case of thalidomide to take the European experience with the drug into consideration.

Of course, that's true. It is tempting to overuse the privilege of hindsight and describe Merrell as an entirely diabolical organization. While its attitude can fairly be assessed as unethical, insensitive and unscrupulous, by the time Merrell submitted its NDA to the FDA, thalidomide was already in wide use in Germany, England, and several other countries. Major concerns regarding the drug's safety were yet to be raised, and no one imagined what unspeakably dreadful harm it could cause in an unborn child.

Still, when Frankie raised her first concerns about its NDA, Merrell's absolute priority *should* have been to lead a thorough investigation into these objections, rather than to push its marketing plans to release the drugs as early as possible for maximum profit.

Before Merrell planned and conducted its study, thalidomide had been submitted to tests by Chemie Grünenthal in Germany and in England, via Distillers. Unfortunately, these tests were pretty much useless: they didn't account for the effect of thalidomide on an unborn child, because you *can't* test for that. Also – and Merrell didn't seem to know this – Distillers itself had very little idea what the properties of thalidomide were; it was as ignorant as Merrell in this respect.

One claim that Merrell was making for the drug – a claim that in fact proved justified – was that you couldn't fatally overdose on it. In Britain, Distillers was promoting its version of thalidomide, Distaval, by emphasizing this particular attribute, even to the extent of running a newspaper ad showing a toddler about to raid a medicine cabinet. The wording of the ad argued that Distaval presented no danger to little children. While this was true if they ingested it after being born, it turned out to be horribly false for children who were exposed to it before birth.

In fact, Distillers – a beverage company that had decided to set up a pharmaceutical marketing wing, then made the disastrous decision to, in effect, license Contergan from Grünenthal and rebrand it as Distaval for sale in the UK – was pretty much in the dark about the real nature of thalidomide.

A little-known letter written on 1 September 1959, from W. P. Kennedy of the Distillers Company (Biochemicals) Limited to Dr Mückter of Grünenthal reveals blatantly, openly, and inadvertently how little Distillers actually knew about the drug it was already marketing widely in the United Kingdom. As Kennedy wrote:

> Dear Dr Müchter,
>
> When we met in Prague, you told me that you hoped to be able to let us have a report of a method for estimating Contergan in urine and the blood. I would be glad to know how this is progressing. The special reason for this is that very soon we are arranging to discuss the drug with a professor of biochemistry and a professor of pharmacology in the hope that they will [be] induced to start some basic work on the drug in their departments. We feel that we do not know enough about the metabolism and pharmacological effects of Contergan and that increased knowledge will lead to wider applications for it.
>
> Did you not also say that you were doing some experiments with radio-active labeling of the Contergan molecule? I am not sure about this, but if I'm correct, I hope you will be able to tell me something of this too – in particular what atom of the molecule you have labeled.

There are probably very few sentences written in the history of medicine – or in the history of science, or indeed in the history of anything – that are more of an understatement than the sentence: 'We feel that we do not know enough about the metabolism and pharmacological effects of Contergan ... .'

That said, the problem of overdose was at the time, and still is, a major danger with sleeping pills such as barbiturates, which can easily cause death if taken in greater quantities than prescribed. These frequently were used at the time by people intent on committing suicide – usually successfully due to the potency of the drug. Under US law, Merrell was required to conduct its own clinical investigation, but it had good reason to believe that nothing unfavorable would emerge from it. In Merrell's view, thalidomide had been sufficiently studied in Germany and England. Thus, the company used the FDA-required study to introduce the drug and create a positive climate for marketing thalidomide in the United States. Even though Merrell had a reasonable basis to believe that its clinical study would not reveal anything new, its use of that study for marketing efforts was a perversion of the Food, Drug and Cosmetic Act.

We now need to ask a vital and thoroughly logical question: why, more than five years after thalidomide had been launched in the West German market, *was* there still such global ignorance of the true nature of this drug?

There were, perhaps, four main reasons why the disastrous effect thalidomide had on unborn children still was not known even at this time. The first was the fundamental fact that by the time a thalidomide-afflicted baby was born, mothers had often forgotten that they'd taken thalidomide at all. Even if they did remember, they had no reason to suspect a link between the tablets and their disabled baby, especially since thalidomide could cause its dire effects even if only one tablet was taken. In practice, most mothers who used thalidomide took more than one tablet, but many mothers only took a few, and by the time their babies were born, they would not attach any significance to the memory of having taken this medicine, especially considering the utter trauma they were suffering after the birth.

Secondly, as we've mentioned, the sheer variety of brand names for thalidomide was a major reason the truth about the drug's harmful effects took so long to become public knowledge globally. Even if a mother *did* remember having taken a particular drug early in the pregnancy and communicated this to her doctor, or if the doctor looked at her prescription history, the variety of brand names made it difficult for doctors working in different countries to communicate about their experience of a particular branded drug.

A third reason the truth about the thalidomide nightmare took so long to come out was the communications technology of the late 1950s and early 1960s – or rather, the lack of it. Abundant, worldwide exchanges of information were not yet part of people's lives. Many people in the early 1960s, even in economically developed countries such as the United States, Britain and West Germany, did not even have telephones in their homes, let alone information technology machines that could communicate with similar machines around the world. Even the very beginnings of the Internet still lay about three decades in the future. In the late 1950s and early 1960s, the nightmarish nature of what thalidomide could do to babies was simply unknown and unshared: individual cases were very much individual nightmares.

Yet perhaps the most important reason it took so long for the truth about thalidomide to come out was the fourth reason: no one really imagined that a drug could cause such disastrous effects on babies. The idea that a drug prescribed for morning sickness could be the culprit required an enormous leap of imagination, and at this point, no one on the planet was prepared to go there.

On 10 November 1960, the last day before Merrell's thalidomide NDA would have led to the licensing of Kevadon unless the FDA objected, Frankie wrote to Merrell and pointed out numerous inadequacies in the NDA. These included insufficient data about chronic toxicity, incomplete detail about both the animal and clinical studies that had been performed, and limited information about the drug's stability. These objections extended the effective date for Merrell to market thalidomide for at least another sixty days, but even more importantly, they served notice on Merrell that the FDA was not going to rubber-stamp Merrell's NDA based on the thalidomide experience in Europe.

Merrell had little or no patience for Frankie's requests for additional information and the delays occasioned by them. In October, Merrell had inquired about who was assigned to review its NDA for thalidomide, as was its right under FDA practice. Thereafter, Merrell engaged in a sustained and determined campaign to truncate review of its NDA not only with Frankie, but with her superiors as well. Merrell initiated over fifty contacts with Frankie during the period when thalidomide was under review. In retrospect, Frankie, with her characteristic reserve and fondness for understatement, observed: 'Whereas other firms had on occasion applied pressure, in no instances was it as severe as with this application'.

The following is a chronology of interactions between Merrell and the FDA, the main counterparty of whom was usually Frankie, during the first five months following the initiation of the thalidomide NDA. This material is supplied by the US Bureau of Medicine, so is written in the first person from the perspective of the FDA. The parentheses are from the source material.

September 12, 1960
The application was submitted.

September 15, 1960
We issued a routine letter of acknowledgment.

October 25, 1960, or sometime later
Murray called Dr Smith to learn what medical officer was reviewing the application.

November 10, 1960
Our letter found the application incomplete and inadequate to demonstrate safety. The chemist's data also were incomplete. The proposed labeling was unsuitable, and inappropriate comments were given insofar as possible.

November 30, 1960

Firm submitted some of the data (on chemistry) to partially complete the application.

December 16, 1960

Murray and Mr. Muhlenpoh met with several of our representatives to submit further data and to present verbal information in support of their application.

December 28, 1960

Mr. Casale submitted additional clinical data: a covering letter from Murray anticipated another conference.

December 29, 1960

Dr Kelsey called Murray to point out a deficiency in the submission of the previous day. Some material was not in duplicate. Murray said this material was intended for her personal information and not for inclusion in the application. Dr Kelsey did not agree with this procedure, so another copy was promised. Dr Kelsey explained the delay and confusion entailed by personal submissions of material. Murray urged her to set a conference date soon and expressed the applicant's hurry to provide for marketing the drug. [Presumably the duplicate material was later submitted; it would be in the duplicate copy of the NDA.]

January 9, 1961

Murray called both Dr Kelsey and Miss Geismar (the chemist reviewing the application). He gave certain information on chemistry and inquired whether certain other data were sufficient: these had not been reviewed but were thought probably sufficient. He asked for an appointment with Dr Kelsey to discuss new proposed labeling. Dr Kelsey agreed to attempt to see him if her schedule permitted. The merits of certain data were also discussed in this telephone call.

January 11, 1961

Murray personally submitted an amendment to Dr Kelsey containing chemical, pharmacological, and clinical data.

January 17, 1961

Revised proposed labeling was submitted together with clinical information. Murray's covering letter requested that he be called if the material were satisfactory so that the applicant might proceed with its plans for production and marketing.

January 17, 1961

Our letter stated that the application was considered withdrawn and resubmitted.

January 25, 1961

Murray called Dr Smith. He said he had tried to phone Dr Kelsey but had learned she would not be available for an indefinite period. Dr Smith confirmed this fact. Murray said the NDA awaited only review of revised labeling which they were waiting to have printed. Dr Smith promised to investigate.

January 31, 1961

Murray called Dr Smith and asked if he had anything to report on Kevadon. Dr Smith said he had spoken to Dr Kelsey about it and had learned that there was more to review than a few labeling changes. Considerable material submitted before our last letter had not yet been reviewed. Murray indicated that the firm would have to postpone its marketing schedule and asked to be called if he could help us.

February 1, 1961

Murray told Dr Kelsey by telephone that 'release' was scheduled for Kevadon on March 6 and wanted to print labeling. Dr Kelsey indicated that she would review the material as soon as possible but explained the press of other matters keeping her busy. (Dr Kelsey's preoccupation with other business is understandable; this was the hearing to suspend the application for Altafur.)

February 15, 1961

Murray called Dr Smith and referred to a recent conversation with Dr Kelsey. He said Dr Kelsey told him the application was probably all right if specified labeling changes had been made, but that review was still pending. Murray spoke of being under pressure to 'get it through' because of the need for preparation for marketing. He said the firm's vice president had advised a trip to Washington, but agreed with Dr Smith that this would be of no use since Dr Kelsey was not available. Dr Smith thought Dr Kelsey would be available after that week.

February 16, 1961

Murray called Dr Kelsey, referred to yesterday's call to Dr Smith, and 'wondered about Kevadon'. Dr Kelsey hoped to get to it the next week. Murray referred to a previous promise to get to it in one day; Dr Kelsey disagreed that such a promise had been made, and Murray decided he probably had misunderstood.

February 23, 1961

Our letter found the application incomplete. We had learned of reports of neurological toxicity from the medical literature. Therefore, data from further animal studies, which were in progress, were needed. Further clinical information was needed.

Eleven

THE BATTLE RAGES

Between September 1960 and November 1961, when the news broke around the world about thalidomide's responsibility for the birth of deformed babies, Frankie and Merrell were locked in what was, on the face of it, a polite battle over Merrell's dissatisfaction with the way Frankie was handling the NDA. In truth, however, Merrell was often not very polite to Frankie, though it is to her credit that she always kept her cool, even under considerable provocation.

As Merrell's self-imposed March 1960 deadline for launching thalidomide into the bloodstreams of pregnant American women came and went, Dr Joseph Murray's dreams of bonuses from the success of thalidomide in the US began to evaporate, and he became increasingly annoyed and frustrated with Frankie.

Merrell's dissatisfaction stemmed not only from her refusal to approve the drug but also from its conviction that Frankie, as a woman, was somehow exceeding her authority in not allowing the male company executives of Merrell to launch on the American market the ten million thalidomide Kevadon tablets they wanted to sell across the nation.

Again and again, we realize that Frankie's memory of what happened is relatively kind to Merrell: it's only when one looks at the actual correspondence between Frankie and Merrell that one realizes how insidious and in many ways unethical Merrell's attempts to get the thalidomide NDA passed really were.

To go once more into further detail than the summary of the first five months of the conflict presented above by the Bureau of Medicine, a handwritten memo by Frankie recalls that on 28 December 1960, she made a call to Murray:

> Advising him that Merrell's local representative had only left one copy of some additional material. Dr Murray claimed this file was meant for my personal attention rather than for inclusion in [the] NDA. So he said he would send an additional copy. I explained to him the delay and confusion entailed by personal submission of material. He urged me to set a conference date in the near future, as they were anxious to market Kevadon, and it would require them to detail their salesmen, etc. I made no commitments.

This was the pattern of the interaction between Merrell and Frankie for the next eleven months; Murray would push, probe, try to persuade Frankie, and try to coerce her, instead of seriously looking into her concerns about the thalidomide NDA. He tried pretty much every stratagem and tactic imaginable, except for actual physical assault and direct bribery, and if he felt these would have facilitated the advent of his dream of selling thalidomide to the United States he might have tried those too. But Frankie was not to be pushed, probed, persuaded, coerced or anything else.

On 30 December 1960, two days after Frankie made this phone call, her husband, Ellis, who had seen some of the supporting evidence for the thalidomide NDA, wrote a memo to his wife with important content relating to her vital work in assessing it. While Ellis did not work with Frankie at the FDA, theirs had always been a marriage founded on a deep and shared love of medical and pharmacological matters. Ellis entitled his memo 'Comment on information concerning Kevadon submitted by W.F. Merrell Co. December 9, 1960'. His most strident comments are these:

A. The section entitled 'Chemical Comparison of Thalidomide and Glutethimide' is an interesting collection of meaningless pseudoscientific jargon apparently designed to impress chemically unsophisticated readers.

(1) There is no conceivable significance in a distinction between 'natural' and 'synthetic'' precursors to a synthetic chemical. In either case the final product is 'unnatural'.

(2) Selection of one chemical difference between two compounds as the 'most important chemical difference' is absurd. What is the 'most important' difference between an apple and an orange?

Ellis went to explain in more technical detail how useless he considered a section of the submission entitled 'Absorption Studies in Rats With C-14 Labeled Thalidomide'. He says: 'the experimental procedure used is either undescribed or inadequate. The data are completely meaningless as presented'. He concludes 'In summary, none of these data is of any value whatsoever, except to demonstrate that all of the drug is not excreted unchanged in the feces'. He goes on to point out: 'in the section 'Pharmacological Comparison Between Thalidomide and Glutethimide' appears a very unusual claim that thalidomide has *no* LD'. As he says, 'No other substance can make *that* claim'. What Ellis means is that *every* substance does have some dosage level that will kill. For example, drinking an extremely excessive amount of water would obviously be fatal, and even chocolate has a fatal dosage level for an adult (a reassuringly high 28 pounds) – assuming anyone could eat even close to that amount and keep it down.

Ellis Kelsey was showing the thalidomide NDA for the piece of amateurishly incompetent drivel it mostly was.

He also goes on to say:

> The last sentence in this section is an almost classical example of the widely used irrelevancy of size-of-dose comparisons between drugs. Weight is never a determinant of activity or toxicity; this is a property of each drug. For example one gram of a great many drugs is very much less toxic (or effective) than one hundredth of a gram of a large number of other drugs. Since this is an elementary concept of pharmacology, I cannot believe this to be honest incompetence.

Ellis's comments on the submission by Merrell made a deep impression on Frankie and put her even more on guard than she already was to Merrell's willingness to try to blind her with science or use dishonest language in order to obtain its much-dreamed-of permission to market its drug. Frankie describes what she regards as 'the next step in the story':

> Probably in late January or early February of 1961 ... my attention was drawn to a letter to the editor by Dr Leslie Florence in *The British Medical Journal* of December 31, 1960, in which he reported peripheral neuritis, a very painful tingling of the arms and feet, in patients receiving the drug thalidomide for a fair period of time. This effect was very severe in some cases and probably not reversible.

Here is the letter to which Frankie refers:

> *Is Thalidomide to Blame?*
> Sir – I feel that four cases which have occurred in my practice recently are worthy of mention, as they may correspond to the experience of other practitioners. They all presented in more or less the same way – each patient complaining of: (1) Marked paraesthesia affecting first the feet and subsequently the hands. (2) Coldness of the extremities and marked pallor of the toes and fingers on exposure to even moderately cold conditions. (3)

Occasional slight ataxia. (4) Nocturnal cramp in the leg muscles. Clinical examination in each case has been essentially negative, and during this time I have not noticed similar cases in my practice. It seemed to me to be significant that each patient has been receiving thalidomide ('Distaval') in a dose of one hundred milligrams at night, the period during which the drug had been given varying from eighteen months [to] over two years. Thalidomide is generally regarded as being remarkably free of toxic effects, but in this instance the drug was stopped. Three of the patients have now received no thalidomide for two to three months, and there has been a marked improvement in their symptoms, but they are still present. The fourth patient stopped taking the drug two weeks ago, and it is therefore too early to assess the effect of withdrawal.

It would appear that these symptoms could be a toxic effect of thalidomide. I have seen no record of interest to learn whether any of your readers have observed these effects after long-term treatment with the drug. I might add that I have found it otherwise to be a most effective hypnotic with no 'morning hangover' effect. It has been especially useful in patients with skin puritus and discomfort.

I am, etc.,

A. Leslie Florence

Turriff Aberdeenshire

Dr Florence was completely right in his suspicions that thalidomide was responsible for the symptoms he had observed. It is now known that thalidomide causes peripheral neuritis in the limbs of adults in much the same way that it causes embryonic limbs to fail to develop properly: by inhibiting blood flow to limbs. Thalidomide also has other effects which even today are not fully understood.

When you saw the heading of Dr Florence's letter, you might have wondered whether the letter might actually have raised the possibility that thalidomide was responsible for deformation of unborn babies. But although that's not the area relating to his suspicions, the very fact that thalidomide caused peripheral neuritis and limb deformities with unborn children might have led Dr Florence to investigate the reactions of any pregnant women patients to whom he had given the drug. There is no record, however, of whether any of his patients had been pregnant when he gave it to them or what the consequences of them having taken thalidomide might have been.

That letter played a vital part in beginning to raise Frankie's suspicions about thalidomide not being the great, side–effect–free wonder drug it was described as. As Frankie remembers:

I was browsing the journal when I read this in late January or early February 1961. The *BMJ* was one of the journals we browsed through. Its format is very amenable to that. When this issue had been published on December 31, 1960, there was a problem with delivery of our journals – I think it was a mail strike – and the journal did not reach us until late January or early February. But the peripheral neuritis did not seem the sort of side effect that should come from a simple sleeping pill. We immediately drafted a letter to the company [Merrell] asking for more information and for more proof of safety. It was apparent this effect might be associated with the use of the drug.

Once Frankie had been alerted to the possibility that thalidomide caused peripheral neuritis – and from the outset she seems to have regarded it as a likelihood – she never totally trusted the thalidomide NDA again.

Then, on 14 January 1961, a follow-up letter was published in *The British Medical Journal* written by Denis Burley of the clinical research department of the Distillers Company (Biochemicals) Limited, London SW1:

Sir – In view of Dr A Leslie [Florence's] letter (December 31, 1954) reporting a possible toxic hazard with the sedative/hypnotic drug thalidomide ('Distaval'), I feel it is important to record here our present information on this aspect gleaned from four years' clinical investigation.

Until recently both animal experimental work and clinical studies have not revealed any significant toxic hazard from thalidomide, but early in 1960 isolated reports ... sent to me from various parts of the country described symptoms and signs suggesting that peripheral neuritis [occurred] in patients receiving thalidomide regularly for periods of six months or more. In some of these cases, because of either inadequate data or the simultaneous use of other drugs, it was impossible to say whether thalidomide was responsible. For mothers, however, we felt satisfied peripheral neuritis could be a toxic hazard, albeit a rare one, and since August of last year information about this had been included in literature supplied with the drug.

The majority of doctors using thalidomide for prolonged periods have observed no adverse reactions, but because of Dr [Florence's] report and the others I have mentioned, we recommend a watch should be kept for changes in the sensation in the peripheries should the drug be given over a period of months.

It is not known for certain whether Frankie read this letter, but she probably did – she was highly vigilant about any reports linking thalidomide with peripheral neuritis. In addition, in view of the diligence which Frankie applied to her professional work, she wasn't impressed that Merrell neglected to mention peripheral neuritis and subsequently even seemed to play down the side effects caused by thalidomide.

Gradually, as more and more evidence about peripheral neuritis being caused by thalidomide appeared worldwide, Merrell's approach to this matter could be described less as playing down this side effect and more as doing its utmost to conceal it. When one looks at the evidence, Frankie's comments in her memoir about this matter seem to be more favorable to Merrell than it deserves.

We later learned that this effect [peripheral neuritis] had been recognized not only at this time, but earlier in Europe, and it was the main reason why the drug had been removed from over-the-counter status in Germany and made a prescription item. (I do not think it was ever sold over-the-counter in

England.) [Frankie is right about this; it never was.] The labeling of the drug by the European companies had carried a warning of a possible side effect of peripheral neuritis, and I believe it was on the label at the time that the application was submitted to us because these side effects are often realized before they are reported in print in journals. Despite this side effect being known in Europe at the time we received the application, communications were poor in those days, and we were simply not aware of this until we had had the drug for about six to eight months. So there was an awareness of this adverse effect before this publication appeared, but not by us.

The crucial point Frankie herself makes about communications being poor 'in those days' is, as we've seen, a major reason why there was such a delay before the truth about thalidomide and its effects on the unborn became public knowledge. As for how Frankie saw Merrell's attitude toward the revelations about peripheral neuritis, this section by Frankie is absolutely vital in setting down the sad story of Merrell's persistence with the thalidomide NDA. She recalls:

We had no way of knowing whether Merrell in general was aware of this problem. They did have representatives overseas, but sometimes the foreign operations of a domestic drug firm are completely separate from those in the United States. Murray claimed that he had noted the letter in the *BMJ* at about the same time we did. It seemed to be a surprise for him. But he did not bring it up with us, although we had several phone calls in this period. I asked him about it, I think, on about the third phone call. He'd evidently been aware of the report, but had not volunteered the information that thalidomide could cause peripheral neuritis.

Frankie also recalls that, as a consequence of the letter she saw in the *British Medical Journal,* there was a meeting involving Frankie, Murray, and Dr Ralph Smith, the man to whom Frankie reported at the FDA. It seems clear from her recollection that it was *she* who brought the *BMJ* letter to the attention of Merrell rather than vice-versa. Subsequently, Frankie also recalls Murray trying to convince her that Merrell had first learned of the toxic side effects of thalidomide only from the December issue of the *BMJ*.

Frankie remarks that if that had been the case, then she thought the intelligence (i.e. information-gathering) was very poor because by the early months of 1961, the problem of peripheral neuritis was already well recognized. As she comments: 'They should have known if they had done their homework, or if contacts had been good between the two continents'.

Frankie herself concedes that the nature of the communications on the question of peripheral neuritis between Merrell in Cincinnati and its European business associates wasn't clear.

On 15 February 1961, Dr Ralph Smith made a handwritten note of a phone call he had received from Murray. The note read:

Dr Murray said that he had talked to Dr Kelsey since last talking to me. She said [according to Murray] that [the] NDA was probably all right if the requested changes in [the] brochure had been made, but she still had to review it. He [Murray] said he was under pressure to get it through in connection with the briefing of their sale force and meeting the schedule for marketing.

He [Murray] said that a trip to Washington had been advised by their vice president. He agreed with me that this would have been of no use since Dr Kelsey was not available.

I said I believed she would be free after this week.

Note the insidious emotional pressure Murray tries to inflict on the FDA and Frankie as he attempts to get Dr Smith to sympathize with his predicament. Dr Smith might have reasonably pointed out that the FDA needed to carry out its legal duty and that Merrell's marketing plans were irrelevant. But Dr Smith was clearly too polite to point this out. However,

Murray's pushiness didn't really deserve politeness. Indeed, a constant theme in the whole Murray–Frankie interaction is the enormous restraint shown by Dr Smith and Frankie in the face of the pressure and emotional blackmail often displayed by Murray.

On February 16, 1961, Frankie wrote this memo by hand:

> Dr Murray called. He said he had spoken to Dr Smith yesterday. He wondered about Kevadon. I said I hoped to get to it next week. He said last time I spoke to him I would get to it next day. I assured him I had never been that optimistic. He agreed he had probably misunderstood me.

Or more to the point, he no doubt hadn't really misunderstood Frankie, but it was temporarily convenient for Murray to pretend he had.

A week later, on 23 February a new version of the thalidomide NDA, which had been submitted to the FDA on 17 January 1961, was declared 'incomplete' by Frankie for 'failing to report animal studies in detail'. Frankie used the announcement of the peripheral neuritis side effect in *The British Medical Journal* as the basis for requesting a complete list of doctors who were investigating the drug in the US (by testing it on their patients) so the FDA could ask these doctors whether any of their patients had reported the peripheral neuritis reaction.

On 28 February 1961, Murray wrote the following letter to Frankie:

> Dear Dr Kelsey,
>
> I have your letter of February 23 concerning our new drug application for Kevadon.
>
> On the basis of our telephone conversation of last week, I assume the comments on the animal studies no longer apply. As we discussed, our agreement was to carry out lifetime studies in rats in support of a possible new drug application for proprietary marketing of Kevadon. Your Pharmacology Division expressed complete satisfaction with the interim data we supplied, and of course, in my letter of January 6, 1961, I agreed to make the results of

the lifetime rat studies available upon their termination. Also, of course, the original submission included showed no effect on microscopic pathology.

Your letter refers to reports on peripheral neuritis which appeared in *The British Medical Journal*. As I indicated, we had contacted the Distillers Company for complete details. We have now received a letter from Distillers discussing this problem, but unfortunately not giving full details. In the interest of saving time, Dr Jones of our medical department and I will visit England next week to obtain firsthand information and to review available case histories.

Promptly on our return, all information will be made available to you.

On 2 March 1961, the FDA commented on Murray's 28 February letter. It is likely that Frankie was the author of this comment:

The firm [Merrell] submitted a letter giving some of the information specified in our letter of February 23 and debating the matter of the further animal studies. It appears that Dr Murray assumed from the telephone conversation of February 23 that pharmacological studies as outlined in letter were not needed but could be submitted later at the end of the lifetime experiment. Further clinical information was promised when it could be obtained in England.

Murray called Frankie to report that, on his recent trip to England, he had found that neurological symptoms did occur with prolonged use of Kevadon. This finding was not of great benefit to Merrell of course. It is not known exactly when this phone call took place; the memo reporting on it was not typed up until 8 January 1962. The call certainly happened in March 1961, and giving Murray time to fly to Britain and return, most likely in the second or third week of March.

Murray, the memo noted, had claimed in the phone call that:

if discovered in time, the effects apparently were reversible. His firm had written their investigators in this country [the US] and had obtained some further reports of toxicity. He [Murray] sought an appointment to discuss proposed labeling. Dr Kelsey informed him that we regard the toxicity of Kevadon as serious.

Murray does at least deserve credit for having reported promptly and accurately to Frankie that thalidomide did cause peripheral neuritis. Where he took a risk, though, was in claiming that 'apparently' the effects of the peripheral neuritis were reversible. It is not known what his basis was for claiming this, and most likely he didn't have a basis at all but was just hoping it might be true. Of course, common sense would suggest that the effect of many drugs is reversible when the patient stops taking them, but that is not always the case. For example, it is certainly not true in the case of many poisons. In Murray's case, his cautious assertion would appear, not for the first time, to simply be wishful thinking.

The FDA's memos about the ongoing interactions proceed as follows:

March 30, 1961

Dr Murray submitted further data and discussed clinical aspects of the application with Dr Kelsey and Miss Geismar. A revision was proposed in the amendment to provide a warning about the neurological reactions. The visitors indicated the toxicity was low in incidence and rapidly reversible. (Brief perusal of one report indicated this was not always the case.) They pressed for a verbal commitment that the application would become effective with the precautionary information in the labeling. Dr Kelsey specified the need for a review of material and indicated that the value of the drug would not warrant untoward reactions. (Dr Kelsey's memorandum of this conference explained some suspicion of a lack of complete frankness by the firm.)

March 30, 1961

Dr Murray and Dr Jones visited Dr Smith following their conference with Dr Kelsey and Miss Geismar. They gave his information verbally about the neurological toxicity, believed the advantages of the drug outweighed the risk, and expressed concern about our delay. Dr Smith offered no commitment, stated the need for serious consideration of the matter, and said we might discuss it with investigators or other experts.

March 30, 1961
Our letter stated that the application was considered withdrawn and resubmitted.

[Handwritten:] *March 30, 1961*
Dr Murray submitted additional data concerned with adverse reactions reported in England, Germany, and the United States. The discussion was on clinical aspects of the NDA only. Some of the submissions were package inserts of the drug distributed by foreign companies. It was noted that the translation of one of the inserts did not coincide with the original. Dr Murray explained that the translation may have been made from an earlier copy of similar type.
Lee Geismar

The next memo was written by Frankie. It is undated but probably was written around the end of March 1961.

Drs. Jones and Murray came in to discuss the Kevadon application in view of their recent visit to England and Germany. They maintained the toxicity incidence was low and rapidly reversible. Brief perusal of a report by Cohen in California indicated this was not always the case. They displayed British and German labeling that draw attention to the toxicity. They kept urging me to say we would pass the drug with similar cautions. I pointed out we would have to study the submitted material in detail before reaching any conclusions, as we felt the field of usefulness of the drug was such that untoward reactions would be highly inexcusable. I had the feeling throughout that they were at no time being wholly frank with me and that this attitude was obtained in all our conferences, etc., regarding this drug. I may have been partly prejudiced by their advanced publicity (*Medical Sciences*, March 25, 1961) in which they featured work by Lester which we indicated was inadequate and in which they compared Doriden and Kevadon chemically after they had previously mentioned they were entirely different drugs, and by their failure to notify us of the British reports of toxicity.

Next, Ralph Smith writes:

The visitors had already discussed with Dr Kelsey the problem of the reports of peripheral neuritis caused by Kevadon. They gave me the following information. The incidence of this effect was estimated to be less than 0.5 per cent. In the United States they had five reports from a total of 2,900 cases. There are reports of twenty-seven cases in England and thirty-four in Germany where the drug has been extensively marketed.

They stated that they believed the advantages of this sedative outweigh the low occurrence of this adverse effect and thought that it would be marketed to the advantage of medicine if attention was called in the labeling to the occasional occurrence of peripheral neuritis. They said that they were concerned about the delay which they were experiencing in placing the drug on the market.

I told them that I could make no prediction as to whether they would obtain an effective new drug application or when it would be. I said that it was a matter for serious consideration and that possibly we might discuss the matter with some of our investigators or other experts.

Murray's endlessly inventive audacity persisted. On 4 April 1961, he wrote to Frankie:

Dear Dr Kelsey:

As we mentioned during our visit to your office last Thursday, we had asked [name of a physician-investigator] to send his case reports on patients treated over a long period of time with Kevadon (thalidomide) to our hotel in Washington. Unfortunately, his letter did not arrive before

I left town, so I am enclosing two copies at this time. You will note that he reports only three cases of tingling and numbness out of more than one thousand patients, and he concludes that the drug is an effective hypnotic characterized by a high degree of safety.

As I indicated during our discussion, we are very much concerned when you mentioned the possibility of hearing more about this or related drugs at the federation meetings and in future publications. We felt we had accurately and adequately defined the limits of the 'peripheral neuritis' problem, and we felt that the material left with you constituted adequate documentary proof of the relative safety of this drug for us as claimed.

In view of the fact that we originally submitted this new drug application approximately seven months ago, I am hopeful that you will be able to review the material we left with you at a very early date. We should greatly appreciate being advised of your decision by telephone as soon as possible.

If it would be possible to make a slight modification in the wording of our dosage statement without causing additional delay, we would prefer to substitute the following in place of the original statement:

> The recommended dose of Kevadon is one tablet (one hundred milligrams). Should morning drowsiness occur, a reduced dose of fifty milligrams (one-half tablet) is usually effective. (Occasional refractory cases may require a second tablet.)

On April 13 and 14 Murray called the FDA, again using the ploy of trying to put them under emotional pressure to help him deal with his own management pressures.

This is the Ralph Smith's memo of the first call:

Merrell's Dr Murray said Dr Kelsey had doubted the need for a new hypnotic. He also said his management questioned whether he was pushing the NDA hard enough, and VP Woodward intended to see FDA Com. Larrick 'if nothing was going to be done'.

Dr Murray stated that in a previous interview with Dr Kelsey, she had doubted the need for a new hypnotic. In answer to this they had compiled material from the literature on side effects of barbiturates including cases of peripheral neuritis. He said that he realized that this was a negative approach.

He also said that his management did not believe that he was pushing this application hard enough and wanted to take a hand in it themselves. Accordingly he said he hoped something could be done soon.

I told him that Dr Kelsey was out of town and that she probably wanted to consult some investigators or experts on the problem before reaching any decisions.

This is Ralph Smith's memo of the second call:

Dr Murray asked if there were any new developments on the Kevadon application. I told him that no decision on it had been reached.

He related that his management thought that he had failed to get the application through by the usual methods and that there should be some pressure exerted. Accordingly, Mr. Woodward, their vice president, intended to see Mr. Larrick if nothing was going to be done. He said that they would like a 'yes' or 'no' decision so that they could prepare to go to a hearing if necessary.

I told him that I couldn't give him a decision at this time since, as I had told him before, I believed that Dr Kelsey wished to talk to some of the investigators.

He mentioned the many months that the application had been under consideration – that early in January Dr Kelsey had suggested only minor label changes – then we had withdrawn and resubmitted the application thus extending the time period. Following this, the matter of peripheral neuritis had come up resulting in their trip to Europe to look into the matter and their report to us on their findings. He also stated that their Canadian application had been cleared before peripheral neuritis was reported. Following this they wrote to the Canadian authorities to add a cautionary statement to the labeling. This proved to be acceptable to them. He also mentioned the three years of distribution in Germany where it was the third largest selling drug on the market and the low incidence of peripheral neuritis in that country.

He said that since no action had been taken since their report on the peripheral neuritis, he believed that Dr Kelsey was avoiding a decision. I told him this was not true since she wanted to investigate further. I also told him that we may be misled about the low incidence of peripheral neuritis since there might have been many occurrences which were not attributed to the drug because it wasn't suspected. It often happened that side effects of drugs were not reported until they had been on the market for some time.

Since there seemed to be little more to be said the conversation ended at this point.

Murray again kept up the pressure, evidently under the impression that if he did so, sooner or later the FDA might give in and his beloved drug would be approved. On 19 April he wrote again to the FDA:

Dear Dr Kelsey:

As you know, we have been very much concerned about the long delay in clearing our Kevadon new drug application. Since you still may feel that the barbiturates are safer for hypnotic use, I am enclosing two copies of a literature search we have had conducted on the side effects of the barbiturates. You are well familiar now with the facts on Kevadon, and I am sure a comparison will show that the balance is heavily in favor of Kevadon.

I am also enclosing two reports of a literature survey on peripheral neuritis showing that this condition is a common side effect and that it almost invariably clears up immediately when the responsible drug is discontinued.

When one considers the tremendous distribution this drug has had in Germany and in England, and the number of long-term patient studies showing no side effects, it becomes obvious that the incidence of peripheral neuritis is exceedingly small. Moreover, the rapidity with which the symptoms of peripheral neuritis clear up is adequately documented by Dr Simpson and others who have worked with the drug. I again want to stress that there is actually no proof thalidomide causes peripheral neuritis. The evidence is circumstantial in that patients with the condition improved upon removal of the drug. While one clinic in Germany recorded nine cases of peripheral neuritis 'due to thalidomide', they frankly stated they see an average of one hundred nonspecific peripheral neuritis cases yearly, and there is no way of telling whether the nine in question might actually have been part of the hundred.

In order that we may intelligently proceed with our market plans, I should like to have you advise me of your final decision on this new drug application some time next week.

On 5 May Frankie wrote to Murray with justified firmness.

Dear Dr Murray,

I very much appreciate your letter of April 4, 1961, concerning the new drug application submitted by the Wm. S. Merrell Co. for thalidomide, Kevadon's tablets.

We agree with your view that the only serious complication with respect to the safety of the drug is peripheral neuritis. The fact is that we do not as yet have sufficient information with respect to this toxic effect of the drug to permit a complete evaluation of its safety. Among other things, we do not have sufficient information to share your conclusion that this toxic effect of the drug is completely reversible. Further, from other reports, it appears that the incidence of peripheral neuritis may be very much greater than suggested in your letter.

It is the responsibility of this Administration to be satisfied that a new drug has been demonstrated to be safe before it may be released for general marketing in the United States. The fact that the compound has been available in other countries for some years has no particular significance except as a source of additional information with respect to the properties of the drug. It will be our purpose to consider any reliable information that can be obtained, particularly with respect to the problem of peripheral neuritis in those areas where the drug has been employed.

On the same day, Frankie wrote another letter to Merrell, responding to his later correspondence. This letter annoyed Murray considerably, though there is nothing in it that is objectively unreasonable.

Gentlemen: We acknowledge the receipt of your communications of April 4, 1961, and April 19, 1961, in further reference to your new drug application for the preparation Kevadon tablets.

In our opinion the application as it now stands is entirely inadequate to establish the safety of Kevadon tablets under the proposed labeling. In particular, the application does not include complete reports of adequate animal studies nor sufficiently extensive, complete, and adequate clinical studies to permit an evaluation of the toxic effects of the drug which have been manifested by reported cases of peripheral neuritis. On the present evidence we cannot regard Kevadon tablets as safe in the sense that its usefulness as a sedative-hypnotic outweighs the toxic effects indicated by the cases of peripheral neuritis. Detailed case reports with adequate follow-up studies will be required to determine whether the condition is reversible. Animal studies should include appropriate neurological studies of the central and peripheral nervous systems.

We have taken appropriate note of your contention that it has not been provided that Kevadon tablets actually cause peripheral neuritis, and the fact that the labeling of the drug proposed in your letter of March 29, 1961, fails to make a frank disclosure that the drug has been found to cause peripheral neuritis, in the consideration of an application for a new drug, the burden of proof that the drug causes side effects does not lie with this Administration. The burden of proof that the drug is safe, which must include adequate studies of all of the manifestations of toxicity which medical or clinical experience suggest, lies with the applicant. In this connection, we are much concerned that apparently evidence with respect to the occurrence of peripheral neuritis in England was known to you but not forthrightly disclosed in the application.

Murray now tried, understandably enough, in view of the response he was getting from Frankie, to go over her head. He called Ralph Smith on 9 May 1961, who subsequently wrote this memo:

Dr Murray referred to our recent letter on this application which was signed by Dr F. O. Kelsey. He said that he considered it somewhat libelous. [Handwritten note:] This referred to the implication that the firm was aware of the peripheral neuritis problem for some time without informing us. He inquired whether the firm [Merrell] was dealing personally with Dr Kelsey in this connection and if so, whether the letter was subject to reconsideration. I told him that the letter should be considered as from the FDA but that irrespective of who signed it, it could be reconsidered if he thought he had sufficient reason that such be done.

Then, on 10 May, Murray and a colleague from Merrell, Robert H. Woodward, met with Dr William H. Kessenich, medical director of the FDA, who filed this memo.

The above were seen in my office on Wednesday, May 10, 1961.

Dr Murray and Mr. Woodward requested an appointment to discuss a new drug problem. Their NDA had been presented in September 1960, and there had been two subsequent submissions, all of which were deemed incomplete and inadequate. Dr Murray and Mr. Woodward felt they had supplied what was sought and in essence asked what they should now do.

The visitors were told that this was a matter that should properly be worked out with the staff of the Division of New Drugs. It seemed that there was in their minds a problem of communication of what deficiencies we felt the NDA presented – a view I am not sure is justified.

We discussed at some length the philosophy of developing and presenting data to support an NDA and in the manner we reviewed the date submitted. This discussion should not have come as anything new to these men, who have regularly had such matters before us. I gave these visitors no specific remedy for the problems of their NDA. An appointment was made for Mr. Woodward and Dr Murray to see Dr Smith and Dr Kelsey of the Division of New Drugs on Thursday, May 11.

So while Kessenich was happy to take the meeting, he put his trust in Frankie and her judgment. Kessenich met his guests and was courteous to them, but quite rightly he made no special effort to help them.

The following day, 11 May 1961, Murray met with Dr Smith, Frankie, and Dr Archer. The following is the FDA memo of the meeting.

He [Murray] asked what could be done to expedite his application. He explained a failure of communications between his company and the European companies regarding neurological toxicity. Dr Kelsey, following this conference, was inclined to accept Dr Murray's statement that he had only learned of the toxicity when he read the *British Medical Journal* of December 1960. We discussed certain points as being ones on which more information was necessary. These included both animal studies and clinical information. It was at this conference that we specified a need for evidence that the drug would be safe during pregnancy. [Handwritten note on original reads: This was based on peripheral neuritis symptoms in adults.] At this time our concern was only on theoretical grounds.

Woodward sent Kessenich a follow-up letter on 11 May.

Dear Dr Kessenich,

The opportunity of discussing with you last Wednesday our specific problem with the Kevadon NDA was sincerely appreciated. I feel, however, that in addition to this specific situation, there was much accomplished in our review of new drug application procedures in general.

This type of interchange is certainly valuable to the manufacturer: and I hope that in the future when and if communications should again be a problem, we will be able to utilize your good offices.

We are proceeding immediately to develop the data necessary to complete the Kevadon application, and Dr Murray will make this available to Dr Kelsey and Dr Smith promptly.

Thank you again for your assistance.

Very truly yours,

Robert H. Woodward

A week later, Merrell decided to send the FDA a copy of one of its own interdepartmental memos.

Interdepartment Memo – the Wm. S. Merrell Co.

May 19, 1961

To: F. J. Murray

From: T. L. Jones

Subject: Incidence of peripheral neuritis in patients receiving Kevadon in the United States

In response to your question as to the number of patients who have taken one hundred milligrams of Kevadon nightly for three months or longer, the total is over eight thousand patients. All of these patients have taken the drug continuously from three months to twenty-four months. The dosage has been one hundred milligrams or greater. A total of six cases of peripheral neuritis has been reported in this group. In two of these cases, the causative factor of the peripheral neuritis is questionable. This has been due to preexisting disease and drug therapy prior to the administration of Kevadon. (The two cases in question are the ones reported by Drs. McHardy and Cohen.)

Clearly, the point of this memo was to try to convince Frankie that the likelihood of a patient who took thalidomide developing peripheral neuritis was very small. But Frankie remained unconvinced of this.

The FDA's record of the interaction with Merrell continues as follows:

May 25, 1961
Dr Murray called Dr Smith and Dr Kelsey to arrange an appointment to bring in more data.

May 31, 1961
Dr Murray submitted an amendment to Dr Kelsey personally containing clinical data. A long explanatory covering letter included, among other things, reference to data in the amendment and previous submissions demonstrating that Kevadon was safe for the fetus when administered to pregnant women. (It should be mentioned that these studies generally were conducted late in pregnancy: I have not determined in this review whether all involved only late pregnancy.)

June 8, 1961
Dr Murray called Dr Kelsey to ask 'how Kevadon was'. He was told the application was in our Division of Pharmacology, and was asked about certain further data.

June 29, 1961
Drs. Murray and Bunde visited Drs. Siegel, Smith, Kelsey, Talbot, and Weiss and Mr. Hauser. [Dr Archer also was present, but this was inadvertently omitted from the memorandum.] This conference was largely on a separate subject, although Kevadon was discussed. The firm conceded some toxicity but pointed out certain advantages. The discussion centered around whether we would ever grant an effective application. We pointed out the need for further specified studies.

July 10, 1961

A manuscript of a paper based upon data previously submitted was received from the firm.

July 19, 1961

An amendment was submitted containing pharmacological data.

July 26, 1961

Our letter stated that the application was regarded as withdrawn and resubmitted.

July 27, 1961

Dr Murray called Dr Kelsey to determine whether we had received certain pharmacological data. We had, but it was not all that was needed. Dr Murray denied memory of the further requirement. A publication on Kevadon toxicity was discussed.

On 27 July Frankie wrote a memo about a call she received from Murray.

Dr Murray called to see if we had received animal absorption data. I said we had but reminded him we had asked for human absorption data. He denied any memory of our request along this line. I drew his attention to the report in *Medical World News* where Ayd reported on Kevadon without mentioning peripheral neuritis.

No doubt this cheered Murray. Frankie was as usual trying to be polite, but she remained convinced that peripheral neuritis was a major side effect of thalidomide.

The following developments then took place. Here, as before, 'we' means the FDA and 'the firm' means Merrell.

July 31, 1961

We received a letter from the firm discussing the paper and data mentioned in the memorandum of telephone call on July 27.

August 2, 1961

We received an amendment pointing out neurological toxicity from barbiturates.

August 10, 1961

The firm wanted to bring in a group of investigators to present their experience with Kevadon. Dr Murray, in a telephone call to Dr Kelsey, suggested holding this conference in a Washington hotel; she told him to contact Dr Kessenich. (Although no document is available regarding the telephone call, Dr Kessenich specified that the conference should be in our own building.)

August 16, 1961

Dr Murray called Dr Kelsey regarding details of the forthcoming meeting with investigators.

August 23, 1961

We received a protocol regarding the forthcoming meeting.

August 25, 1961

Dr Murray called Dr Kelsey about the conference, which was to be held on September 7, 1961.

Merrell now wanted another meeting with the FDA, and a meeting was granted on 7 September 1961.

Dear Dr Kelsey: In connection with our proposed meeting on Kevadon to be held in Washington on September 7, I am enclosing four copies of a list of investigators who are planning to attend. We have not been able to contact Dr Lasagna, since he is out of the office until after Labor Day, but we will be in touch with him as soon as he returns and I am still hopeful that he will be able to attend.

Sincerely yours,

F. Jos. Murray

P.S. I will be accompanied by the following from Merrell:

    T. L. Jones, MD, associate director of clinical research

    J. N. Premi, MD, Canadian medical director

    E. F. Van Maanen, PhD, director of biological sciences.

The following is Frankie's memo of this meeting.

September 7, 1961

Our representatives met with Drs. Murray and Jones together with a group of clinical investigators that the firm had brought in. (I do not find a list of names, but our representatives included Drs. Kessenich, Siegel, Smith, Kelsey, Nestor, and Archer.) The investigators presented their experience with Kevadon. This included evidence that the drug is effective, has certain advantages over other hypnotics regarding safety, does not cause neurological reactions, and some evidence but not conclusive evidence that the reactions are necessarily reversible. There was only a little evidence that the drug would be harmless to the fetus if given during pregnancy, and this evidence was not adequate. (Our concern with this matter of pregnancy was still only on a theoretical basis at that time.)

Well, maybe so, but it is clear that ever since Frankie had begun to suspect back in early 1961 that Kevadon might cause problems to the unborn child, the possibility that it might be a threat to the fetus never seems to have left her mind for long, at least not as far as her professional duties at the FDA were concerned.

The following are the FDA's summary of developments in the Merrell-FDA contact during September 1961.

September 12, 1961

We received a letter from the firm proposing labeling revision regarding dosage and adverse effects.

September 13, 1961

Our letter found the application still incomplete. In particular, we were awaiting receipt of the data relative to the safety of the drug presented orally in the conference of September 7, 1961.

September 18, 1961

Dr Murray called Dr Kelsey to determine what additional data were needed. She told him we needed the toxicity data reported at the recent conference.

September 26, 1961

Dr Murray called Dr Smith to ask whether he could predict when the application would become effective. He wanted the drug on the market by the middle of November and, in this case, they should commence printing the labeling early in October. He discussed a revised warning statement in the labeling and stated that case reports mentioned at the recent conference would be submitted in a day or so. Dr Smith offered no prediction; he checked with Dr Kelsey and informed Dr Murray that other labeling changes would be necessary including advice against administration in pregnancy. (Our concern with pregnancy still was on theoretical grounds; convincing evidence of safety had not been submitted – we still had no direct evidence of toxicity in this regard.)

The telephone call then was switched to Dr Kelsey. Dr Murray tried to get a deadline for 'release' of Kevadon. She repeated Dr Smith's statements about labeling. Dr Murray wondered if he could record labeling changes by telephone and then print labeling for the October deadline (to get the product on the market by Christmas) or bring the labeling in for an okay. Dr Kelsey explained that this procedure was unsatisfactory and rejected it. Summary of Substance of Contact:

Dr Murray asked me if I could predict when this application would become effective. He said that they wished to go on the market by the middle of November and in this case they should commence printing the labeling during the first week of October. He said that following our conference with the investigators, Dr Kelsey had advised that there should be a change in the warning statement in the labeling and that he had also been informed that the application was incomplete until we had received case reports of neuritis which were mentioned at the meeting. He said that these would be submitted in a day or so. I told him that I could not predict when the application would be made effective and I doubted that Dr Kelsey would be able to do so. After checking with Dr Kelsey, I informed him that other changes in labeling were required in connection with exclusion of use in pregnant women and also reference to objective changes in cases of peripheral neuritis. I advised him to talk to Dr Kelsey in this connection if he wished to discuss it in detail. The call was transferred to Dr Kelsey.

Murray just doesn't give up! He continues pushing, cajoling, and using emotional blackmail whenever he thinks it might work, and if that fails simply demanding to know when Kevadon will become licensed. There is something of black comedy about these interactions, or at least about the way Murray conducts himself toward the FDA. It's only when one reflects on what was really at stake here that the black comedy aspect of the interactions vanishes in the harsh daylight of reality.

September 29, 1961
We received revised labeling and additional data, including information on administration during pregnancy, but essentially late pregnancy.

October 2, 1961
We received a letter correcting an accidental omission from the proposed labeling received September 29.

October 19, 1961

We received a further submission relating to the neurological reactions.

October 23, 1961

Dr Jones talked with Dr Nestor by telephone to obtain suggestions of who would be good investigators to study Kevadon in children.

November 2, 1961

The firm submitted revised labeling discussed in a recent telephone conversation with Dr Kelsey.

Further published data were promised by the covering letter.

November 7, 1961

Our letter stated that the application was considered withdrawn and resubmitted.

November 13, 1961

National Drug Co. (which had a similar application) submitted a publication on the usefulness of the drug on behalf of Merrell.

November 15, 1961

We received a submission containing papers and translations from the literature and commentaries on these papers. The letter refers also to a submission of samples and to an authorization for inspection of the premises of another firm as required by current regulations.

This was the last record of contact before the bombshell hit.

Here is the bombshell. It is not known for certain who wrote this particular memo, but it is probable that the author was Frankie – on this occasion writing about herself in the third person.

November 30, 1961

Dr Murray called Dr Kelsey and informed her that the drug had been withdrawn from the German market because of recent reports of congenital abnormalities associated with use of the drug in pregnancy. He expressed hope that the association would prove to be only coincidental. Dr Kelsey pointed out that recent reports indicated the incidence of neurological reactions was higher than previously believed. We questioned the safety of the drug in view of its proposed use.

One yearns for a recording of this phone call, but no such recording exists, apparently. Was Murray apologetic and contrite? One wishes he had been, but somehow we doubt it.

The remaining summary records of the interaction are below.

December 27, 1961

Our letter found the application incomplete in the absence of data relative to the deformities in newborn babies.

March 8, 1962

We received a letter from the firm requesting withdrawal of the application.

March 14, 1962

Our letter acknowledged the withdrawal of the application.

April 11, 1962

Our letter inquired whether Kevadon was still undergoing investigational use. If so, we wanted information on what had been done to warn physicians of its toxic potentialities. We asked what measures were taken by the company to inform physicians of the association between fetal abnormalities and ingestion of Kevadon by mothers during pregnancy, at the time the association first became known to the firm. We also asked for a complete and up-to-date list of all physicians who were supplied with the drug for investigational purposes.

The battle that raged between Murray and Frankie from September 1960 to November 1961 is not, to put it mildly, the proudest chapter in the history of the United States pharmaceutical industry. It is, on the other hand, the proudest chapter in the history of the FDA, at least so far.

By early 1961, fortunately for the mothers and unborn children of the United States, Frances Kelsey had ceased to be convinced by anything about Merrell, whether it was its 'evidence', its NDA, or its executives. Frankie had been on her guard from the beginning due to her professional conscientiousness. By late January or early February 1961, Frankie was unquestionably worried that thalidomide could cause birth deformities. In her memoirs, she mentions reading a publication about peripheral neuritis at that time that first led her and the FDA to wonder about the effect of thalidomide on embryos.

Murray had by now become thoroughly aware of Frankie's concerns that thalidomide might harm unborn children. He wrote to Kessenich that he would 'as requested by Dr Kelsey provide information that would show that thalidomide would not harm unborn babies'.

This 'information' was furnished by a Dr Ray O. Nulsen of Cincinnati. Nulsen is a somewhat shady character in our story. At the time, no one gave Frankie any detailed information about exactly who Nulsen was or how he operated.

In fact, Nulsen had very little training in obstetrics at all.

Later, in a subsequent legal case between the FDA and Merrell, in which the FDA attempted to show that Merrell had behaved illegally, Nulsen admitted under cross-examination that he had not actually written the article. He said that it had been penned by Dr Raymond C. Pogge, the director of Merrell's Department of Medical Research. Nulsen also admitted he had never seen many of the references cited in the article, nor had he kept a detailed record of the number of pills he had received from Merrell or how many he had given his patients. When asked during the hearing if he had any record of his report, Nulsen replied, 'No, it was all verbal'.

As Margaret Truman says in her book *Women of Courage* (1976):

> In short, the study was a fake. Yet Murray presented it to Kelsey as clinical data proving Kevadon was safe for the unborn. Thanks to her experience in pharmacology, Kelsey was unimpressed, even though she was unaware the study was fabricated. She pointed out to Murray that it only dealt with women who had taken the drug for the last three months of pregnancy; the fetus was most sensitive in the first three months.

Whether Merrell's behavior amounted to cunning combined with great presumption and almost complete selfishness or it crossed the border into definite illegality is ultimately a matter of opinion. But whatever you think of it, Merrell unquestionably seems to have forgotten, in its push for status and profits, that a pharmaceutical company is in existence to serve people, not the other way around.

A memo written by Frankie on 26 September 1961, provides final and convincing evidence of her concerns about the use of thalidomide in pregnancy, though of course we know by now that this had been something on her mind since May of that year. We have already quoted this memo in the Prologue, but it is so important that it deserves to be quoted here again, in its proper chronological place.

> Murray of Merrell called to try and get a deadline set for release of Kevadon. I explained I was concerned about the use of the drug in pregnancy because of the possible effect on a fetus and the lack of mention of objective findings in peripheral neuritis. He [Murray] wondered if he could record changes by phone and then print up the brochures for the October deadline (to get product on market by Christmas) or bring them in and have me okay them. I said neither would be acceptable as misunderstandings inevitably result and that he should submit the materials through the usual channels. I said we would get to it as soon as possible but could give no definite commitment.

Given what was subsequently discovered about thalidomide, there is something macabre in this fresh example of the extreme pushiness of Murray's behavior. He tries to get past Frankie's extremely reasonable objections and reservations by phoning her with some information and making clear that he wants to get the product to market by Christmas 1961, presumably as a Christmas present for the moms of the United States.

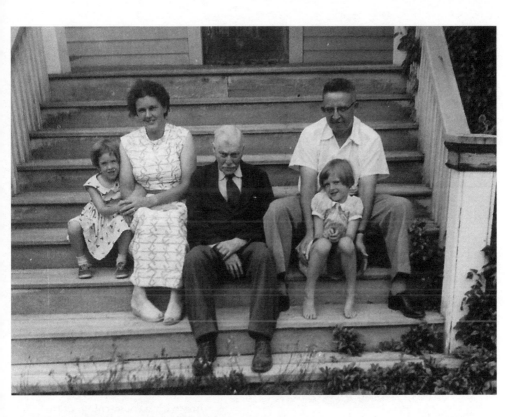

Frances Kelsey and her family. (Authors' collection)

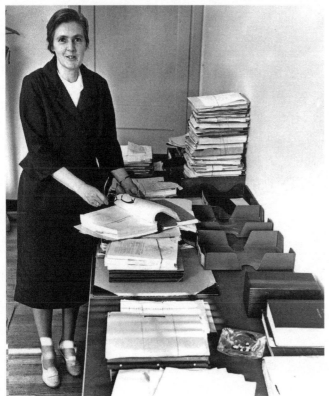

Dr Frances O. Kelsey, pictured here in the 1960s, spent most of her career at the FDA overseeing scientific investigations of drugs. (US Food and Drug Administration)

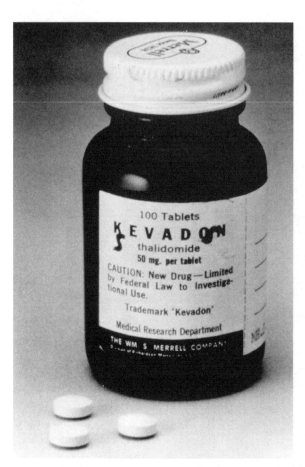

The US name for the drug was Kevadon. (US Food and Drug Administration)

Another more recent brand of thalidomide available in the 2000s, now with stark warnings of the implications for pregnant women and their unborn babies. (Wikimedia Commons/Stephencdickson)

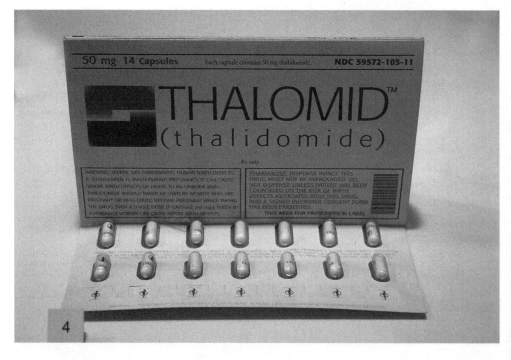

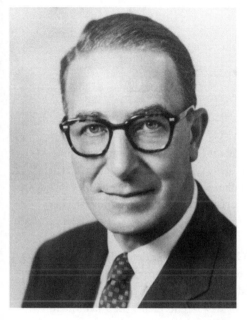

At a time when Carey Estes Kefauver was being accused of increasing government interference in doctor and patient freedoms and threatening the pharmaceutical industry as a whole, the thalidomide scandal helped usher through his Kefauver–Harris Drug Amendments of 1962, which made it compulsory for drug manufacturers to prove the effectiveness and safety of their products before FDA approval, increased the trustworthiness of drug marketing and limited the profits made from cheap new drugs. (US Food and Drug Administration)

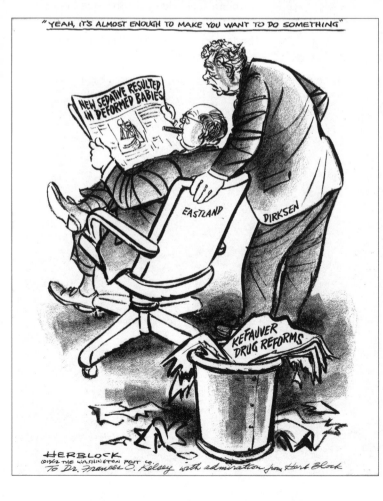

"YEAH, IT'S ALMOST ENOUGH TO MAKE YOU WANT TO DO SOMETHING"

NEW SEDATIVE RESULTED IN DEFORMED BABIES

EASTLAND

DIRKSEN

KEFAUVER DRUG REFORMS

HERBLOCK
©1962 THE WASHINGTON POST CO.
To Dr. Frances O. Kelsey with admiration from Herb Block

Senators James Eastland and Everett Dirksen were among the many who opposed Senator Estes Kefauver's attempts to reform drug regulation in the early 1960s – at the same time as children around the world were suffering the crippling effects of thalidomide. (US Food and Drug Administration)

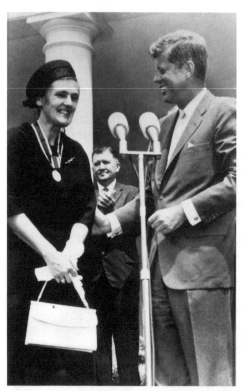

President John F. Kennedy presents the President's Award for Distinguished Federal Civilian Service to Dr Frances Kelsey in August 1962. (US Food and Drug Administration)

US President John F. Kennedy signing the 1962 Drug Amendments to the 1938 Food, Drug, and Cosmetic Act. The FDA's implementation of the new requirements the amendment introduced, upheld by the Supreme Court, revolutionized the drug supply of the US in the decades to follow. (US Food and Drug Administration)

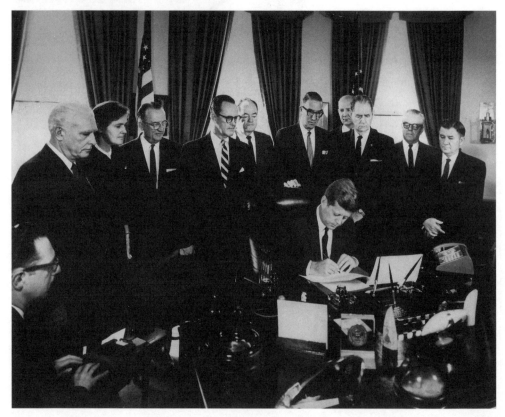

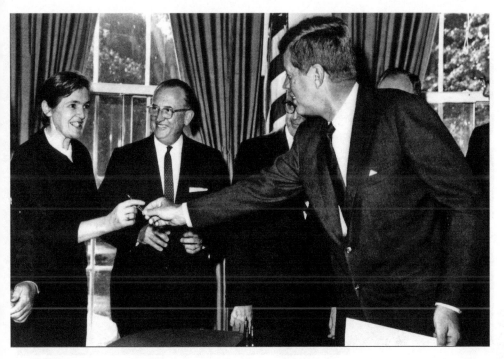

After signing the Kefauver–Harris Drug Amendments on 10 October 1962, President Kennedy presented a pen to those observing the momentous event, including Dr Frances O. Kelsey. (US Food and Drug Administration)

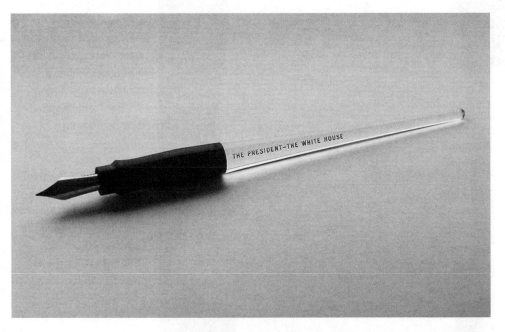

The pen presented to those who observed the signing of the 1962 drug amendments. (US Food and Drug Administration)

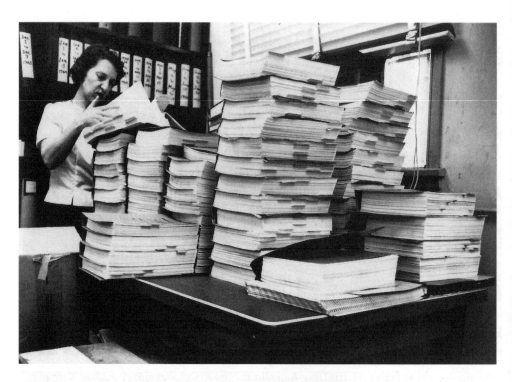

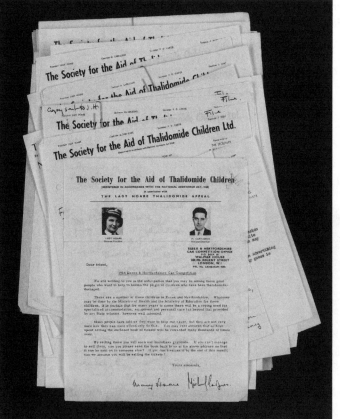

Chemist Lee Geismar, who was part of the team that reviewed the new drug application for thalidomide in the early 1960s, is shown some years later poring over several volumes of another application. (US Food and Drug Administration)

The Society for the aid of Thalidomide Children was set up in the UK to try to help victims of the thalidomide disaster. (The Society for the Aid of Thalidomide Children/Wellcome Collection)

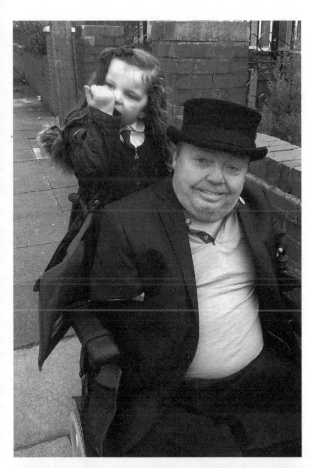

Thalidomide victim Kev Donnellon takes a walk with his daughter Daisy on a sunny spring afternoon. Kev's mother took five tablets of the UK brand of thalidomide, Distaval, for morning sickness in 1961. (Authors' collection)

On September 15, 2010, Commissioner Hamburg presented Frances Kelsey with the first Frances Kelsey Award at a ceremony held at the FDA's White Oak headquarters in Silver Spring, MD. (US Food and Drug Administration)

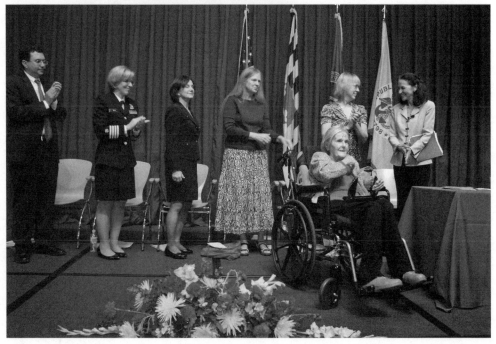

Twelve

AFTERMATH

In her memoir, Dr Kelsey says this of the call Murray made to her on 30 November 1961, informing her that thalidomide was being withdrawn:

> I remember very well when he called and told us about the information he had received from Germany, possibly linking the drug with birth defects. I was – I admit it – very surprised. This is what we had been wanting to make sure would *not* happen with the drug and yet it clearly had.

Once more, Frankie refrains from being vitriolic in ascribing blame toward Merrell. As always she is calm and reasoned in what she says. As she remarks:

> Our objections, as I have pointed out, were really on theoretical grounds, largely based on the fact that there was no evidence that it [thalidomide] was safe. Until we had such evidence we had to question the safety. We received further information from two FDA officials who were in Germany at approximately the time the news came out. They wrote a report on what

they had found. Merrell notified us that they were discontinuing clinical trials with the drug in the United States until they got further information concerning these preliminary reports from Germany on birth defects. So, in essence, we waited for further information, and we did get some in the form of literature reports.

So what exactly had happened? How had thalidomide's disastrous side effects – teratogenicity and peripheral neuritis – finally been identified?

What had occurred is that doctors in Europe had finally reached a consensus that the cause of the deformities in babies must be thalidomide. At that point, enough doctors had looked into what drugs they had prescribed their patients.

Dr William McBride played a major role in ending the thalidomide nightmare. He published a letter in British medical journal *The Lancet* in December 1961 that noted a large number of birth defects in children of patients who had been prescribed thalidomide. As a result of his vital work, ten years later Dr McBride was awarded a medal and prize money by the prestigious L'Institut de la Vie, a French institute that focuses on addressing 'matters connected with the preservation and conservation of life'.

In 1971, McBride established Foundation 41 with the prize money, which was a Sydney-based medical research foundation concerned with the causes of birth defects. It was Dr McBride, working with Dr P.H. Huang, who proposed that thalidomide caused malformation by interfering with the DNA of the dividing embryonic cells. Later on, this finding stimulated experimentation which showed that thalidomide could, in some cases, have positive effects on certain illnesses involving unwanted and malignant tumors, including some forms of leprosy.

Dr McBride was based in Australia and ministered to many patients who had taken Distaval that Distiller had distributed in Australia. As it happened, the first patient to whom Dr McBride had prescribed thalidomide gave birth to a healthy child, even though the patient herself had suffered from severe vomiting after taking the drug. This means that by the time she took the drug, her pregnancy was advanced enough for her unborn child to withstand the effects of thalidomide.

However, three other babies born at the same hospital, Crown Street Women's Hospital in Sydney, which was once the largest maternity hospital in New South Wales, Australia, were not so lucky. On 4 May 1961, McBride attended the birth of baby Wilson. The baby had radial aplasia (missing radius bones in the forearm) and bowel atresia (blockage). Baby Wilson died a week later. On 24 May 1961, McBride attended the birth of another baby who had malformations very similar to those of the Wilson baby, and on June 8 a third baby was born with similar defects. These two babies also died not long after birth.

At the start of a long weekend holiday in June 1961, McBride took home the hospital records of the three babies. He knew very little about teratology (the study of birth defects) and, like most physicians, had hardly ever seen any birth defects during his entire career.

Nor could he find very much in medical literature. He did however read material from the 1960 CIBA symposium on birth defects and possible environmental contamination, and it was clear that this symposium had given attendees the take-home message that drugs could cause birth defects. This led McBride to look at what drugs had been prescribed to the babies' mothers and to subsequently find that the mothers had all taken Distaval. At this point, Dr McBride remembered reading a letter to *The British Medical Journal* from Dr Leslie Florence, the letter we've already quoted, suggesting that long-term use of thalidomide might cause nerve damage – which meant that it was not an entirely harmless drug, regardless of what Distillers was telling him.

By the end of that long weekend, McBride was convinced that the cause of the birth defects in the children who had died was the Distaval their mothers had taken. A couple of days later, he met with a Dr Newlinds at the Crown Street Women's Hospital. Newlinds agreed that McBride's observations made sense, and that very day thalidomide was removed from the hospital's pharmacy. McBride telephoned Distillers and told a representative his conclusions. As for the hospital, it began tests on the effect of thalidomide on mice and guinea pigs.

What happened next is not clear. Certainly, Distillers did not simply pull the drug from the marketplace, which is what it should have done. It was not sufficiently convinced by McBride's warning to do so and, as one might expect, Distillers was making so much money from thalidomide that it was reluctant to acknowledge these concerns. Belief, after all, is often dependent on how much one wants to believe something in the first place. Distillers didn't have a strong incentive to believe that thalidomide was unsafe.

Dr McBride later insisted – and still insists – that on Wednesday, 14 June 1961, he sent a paper to *The Lancet* in London, recording his findings that thalidomide was causing birth defects in Australia. Dr McBride says that his paper was returned on 13 July with a cover letter informing him that *The Lancet* had rejected it for publication. However, it is known that *The Lancet* recorded all submissions, and the magazine has repeatedly said that it has no record of receiving Dr McBride's paper. In addition, Dr McBride has never been able to produce either his original paper, or the reply from *The Lancet*. Obviously if the paper had been published in July 1961, an enormous amount of suffering might have been prevented. We can't think of any reason why Dr McBride would have imagined sending the paper if he had not.

In the summer of 1961, Dr McBride began to doubt that Distaval really had caused the childhood deformities and the problems which had led to the deaths of three babies. In the studies at Crown Street Women's Hospital, none of the animals that were fed thalidomide during pregnancy had delivered malformed offspring. As we now know, this was due to the fact that animals other than primates are not especially vulnerable to the effects of thalidomide. However, Dr McBride was not aware of this at the time.

Also, there hadn't been any other malformed babies born at Crown Street hospital since June, even though many mothers who delivered babies that summer had taken Distaval during pregnancy. The explanation for this is, of course that these women had taken Distaval at a time in their pregnancy when their babies had grown enough not to be affected by it. Unfortunately, it hadn't been discovered yet that thalidomide's effects varied drastically depending on the stage of pregnancy in which the drug was taken.

Naturally enough, Dr McBride began to question his former findings. But his doubts ended in September 1961, when two more babies with thalidomide problems were born at Crown Street hospital. At this point, McBride, who had regained confidence that his hypothesis was correct, once again contacted Distillers. The nightmare was nearly over, though not quite.

Meanwhile, in Germany, despite Chemie Grünenthal's usual efforts to prevent, by any means, its marketing of thalidomide from being constrained, the drug was finally placed under prescription. This action was triggered by unassailable reports of thalidomide causing permanent nerve damage; it was often the case that peripheral neuritis caused by thalidomide was irreversible even if the patient stopped taking the drug. As we've seen, this was something that Frankie had already noted.

Apart from peripheral neuritis, the potential thalidomide had for causing other kinds of damage was still unknown. Grünenthal had ignored the innumerable cases of peripheral neuritis for as long as it could. Because of the resulting negative publicity, the company had lost some market share. One of its motivations for putting the drug under prescription was that it expected it would cause its market share to increase again, now that it had addressed the issue of peripheral neuritis. It hoped that better times were around the corner and was oblivious to the nightmare about to unfold.

Now a physician called Widukind Lenz comes into the story.

Lenz (1919–95) was a German pediatrician and medical geneticist. In 1961, he was one of the first in Germany to recognize and alert the world to the dangers of thalidomide syndrome, and the high risks associated with taking the drug during pregnancy.

From 1937 to 1943, Lenz studied medicine, and was also a group leader in the Hitler Youth, as well as a member of the National Socialist German Students' League and of the SA. However, we need to remember that, at that time in Germany, these sinister factions were all part of the Establishment, and it was normal for Germans to belong to them. After his medical training, from 1944 to 1948, Lenz was employed as a doctor in Luftwaffe hospitals and subsequently in a prisoner-of-war camp in England.

After studying biochemistry in Göttingen and medicine in Kiel, he became chief physician of the Eppendorfer Kinderklinik in 1952. A good-looking, bespectacled fellow with a subdued, thoughtful manner, Lenz was entirely devoted to his patients.

In every respect Lenz was a thoroughly good German. He knew about the growing epidemic of deformed babies being born in West Germany, but he had no idea what could be causing it. Lenz made the heroic decision to study the incidence of birth defects around Hamburg in the two years before 1961. This was not a trivial job in the days before computers.

Lenz, astonishingly, went through *all* of Hamburg's approximately 212,000 birth records from 1930 to 1955. In all that time he found *just one case* of phocomelia. Then, suddenly, he found that, in the twelve months prior to the beginning of his investigation in 1961, there had been eight cases of phocomelia among the 6,420 babies born in Hamburg hospitals.

Lenz became obsessed by what could possibly have caused this epidemic. He came across a paper by a Dr H.R. Wiedemann that described twenty-seven more cases of phocomelia around Kiel and raised the issue of whether one of the newer drugs might be responsible, without actually mentioning thalidomide as a potential culprit. Wiedemann, however, did propose that the malformations he had noted in babies followed a specific pattern that could be described as a syndrome.

Spurred on by reading this paper, Lenz began interviewing mothers of malformed children. Initially, he didn't specifically ask about drugs, but during one of his interviews in November 1961, a woman in Hamburg told him that she had taken thalidomide during her pregnancy.

This lady had experienced peripheral neuritis. She had also been very concerned about her baby. It was this which made Lenz, who was only too well aware of the enormous success of the German-branded version of thalidomide, to wonder whether Contergan itself might have been involved. He called several other physicians, expressed his concerns and asked them if they would make inquiries.

The next day Lenz interviewed several other women who had delivered malformed children, this time asking them specifically about drug use. Four more of them remembered having taken thalidomide during their pregnancy. One of them actually told him that she hadn't originally mentioned Contergan to him during the first interview because it seemed insignificant to her.

Then Lenz had an epiphany that convinced him that all his suspicions were justified. Lenz interviewed a lady who had delivered a malformed child. He then spoke to her doctor, who emphatically told Lenz that he had not prescribed Contergan to this patient but instead had prescribed a drug called Doriden, which does not cause infant malformations. Lenz, however, examined the prescription slip, which was still available, and found a note written by the doctor – who had evidently forgotten what had happened. The note read: *Doriden not available. Replace with Contergan.*

Lenz had placed notices in some newspapers asking mothers who had given birth to deformed infants to come forward. One of those notices was seen by Anneliese Warren, the German wife of a Canadian military officer serving at the military base in Soest.

When Lenz met Anneliese, she displayed a little emotion as she welcomed Lenz and his lawyer friend Karl Schulte-Hillen (who was there because he had a car and Lenz did not). She was obviously a woman of great courage, Lenz later recalled, 'She was so young and innocent'. Early in her pregnancy, Anneliese had been given some medicine for nausea by a doctor located outside the Canadian base.

Her baby, when it was born, had required immediate surgery because of a stomach malformation. The little lad was also afflicted with unnaturally short arms that only had four fingers on each hand, and feet that seemed to be attached to the hips. This was the first time Lenz had heard of lower-body phocomelia as a potential consequence of a mother taking thalidomide.

By the middle of November 1961, Lenz had learned of a total of fourteen cases of birth defects in which the mother had beyond question taken thalidomide. He phoned Dr Mückter at Grünenthal and expressed his suspicions and concerns about the effect of thalidomide on unborn children. Lenz told Mückter he believed that Contergan should be withdrawn immediately from the market and that 'every day the drug remains on the market was in effect a deliberate experiment in human teratology'. Lenz reported that Mückter did not seem especially impressed about the information and was even 'nonchalant' about it. So the next day Lenz followed up with a letter to Grünenthal expressing his concerns. Lenz was absolutely unequivocal in what he said:

> Every month's delay in clarification means that fifty to one hundred horribly mutilated children will be born.

What was Grünenthal's response? It was to ignore him completely. But fortunately, truth cannot be suppressed for long by commercial greed and indifference. As Stephens and Brynner point out in *Dark Remedy*, Thursday, 16 November 1961, was a historic day in the early story of thalidomide.

Pretty much at the same time Lenz was writing to Grünenthal about his fears, Dr William McBride was in Australia meeting with H.O. Woodhouse, assistant sales manager at Distillers, expressing his concerns about Distaval. McBride also wrote again to *The Lancet,* and this time there was no doubt at all that the journal had received the letter, for it was printed the following month.

Two days later, on Saturday, 18 November 1961, Lenz attended a meeting of the pediatricians' association in Sydney, where two doctors – Dr Kosenow and Dr Pfeiffer – presented a paper on the causes of birth defects. After they made their presentation, Lenz stated in public for the first time that 'a certain substance' recently introduced in the West German market was responsible for the current epidemic.

Even then Lenz refrained from naming the drug publicly, but after the meeting a pediatrician approached him and asked him whether or not the drug was Contergan. The pediatrician explained that he and his wife had a malformed child and his wife had taken it. Lenz replied that Contergan was indeed the suspect drug, and before the end of the meeting most of the doctors who attended the event knew that thalidomide was the drug Lenz had been speaking about.

The following day, Sunday, 19 November, three representatives from Grünenthal, including the company's legal adviser, came to see Lenz. The matter was seen as so urgent that the Hamburg Health Authority also attended the meeting. The Grünenthal executives threatened to take legal action against Lenz for what they considered to be an unjustified attack on their company, but by that point the Hamburg Health Authority was more concerned about mothers and their babies than about Grünenthal's obsession with its own commercial success. They asked Grünenthal to withdraw the drug voluntarily from the West German market, but the company refused. The following day, it sent out about 70,000 promotional leaflets to doctors across West Germany declaring that Contergan was a safe drug. Later in the same week, Lenz met once more with Grünenthal representatives, but this time he also invited Schulte-Hillen.

However, the Grünenthal executives refused to continue the meeting while Schulte-Hillen was there, even though their own lawyer was present. Reluctantly, Schulte-Hillen left the meeting. The Grünenthal executives then attacked Lenz and his evidence of fourteen cases. They insisted that his evaluation was not statistically sound. Fortunately, the health authorities were very impressed with Lenz's report and not pleased with Grünenthal's attack on his statistics. They told Grünenthal that Contergan should now be withdrawn from the market and that if Grünenthal did not do this voluntarily, the drug would be banned.

The following day Grünenthal's executives met in their office to examine Lenz's descriptions of the fourteen cases of extremely rare birth defects, and his conclusion that these defects had coincided with the use of thalidomide. They also had in front of them a German translation of the letter which Dr McBride had written to Distillers. Together these documents were evidence enough for any rational person, but rational argument was not always a feature of the activities of Chemie Grünenthal.

Some of the executives present at the meeting were by now convinced that thalidomide had to be withdrawn from the West German market. A pharmacologist at Grünenthal, Dr Herbert Keller, who was relatively inexperienced, later said:

> A teratogenic effect simply never occurred to me. It never occurred to anyone at Grünenthal. I felt like a bus-driver who has run into a group of children and has killed and injured many of them.

There is no evidence that any similar level of remorse was ever expressed by other executives at Grünenthal. As for Mückter, not for the first time, he dug in his heels. Despite overwhelming evidence that the drug on which he had founded the success of his entire career was causing horrific malformations in unborn children, he still refused to take it off the market. In one of the most powerful passages of their book *Dark Remedy*, Stephens and Brynner say:

> It is impossible to resist wondering why he would not agree to a complete withdrawal of the drug, given all that he knew by then. Did he truly believe these birth defects were isolated anomalies, statistical flukes? Or was he, like the army he had served seventeen years earlier, soldiering on in the face of

certain defeat, with a similar contempt for the value of human life, out of loyalty to the shareholders?

Stephens and Brynner go even further, commenting:

That seems like a stretch. But one has to note that, throughout the preceding six months, an even greater moral conflict between individual responsibility and blind loyalty was the leading topic of conversation: the trial of Adolf Eichmann had been broadcast worldwide on television since April with a rapt and deeply divided audience in Germany. Eichmann testified personally about his central role in the Holocaust, at times boastfully taking credit for the Final Solution and the deaths of millions; nonetheless, to every criminal charge, he pleaded not guilty.

They then add:

The trial in Jerusalem revived debates in Germany that had lain dormant since the Nuremberg trials fifteen years earlier. In fact, Eichmann, the architect of Nazi genocide, retained the same defense attorney who represented Goering, Ribbentrop, and Hess. More significantly, Eichmann resorted to the same defense: he'd only obeyed orders. The implication – that individuals have no moral responsibility beyond obedience to their chain of command – was at the core of the banality of Eichmann's evil, in Hannah Arendt's enduring phrase. Ultimately, Mückter and the other manufacturers of thalidomide resorted to a similarly callous courtroom defense. In any case, throughout the time that Eichmann stubbornly insisted upon his innocence in the slaughter of millions, Mückter was fighting 'to the bitter end', to vindicate thalidomide and to defend the rights of the company.

As for Adolf Eichmann, he was hanged by the State of Israel on May 31, 1962, evidently going to his grave still believing that he was only following orders. But of course sometimes a human being is psychologically unable to accept the level of evil to which he or she has stooped.

Whether or not you agree with the comparison drawn by Stephens and Brynner – that Mückter's denial of the truth about the dangers of Contergan somehow relates to Nazism – what is incontestable is that, for West Germans who had survived the war, the allied bombings and the economic 'year zero' (the year after the war ended, when Germany was all but completely destroyed), their country's success in rebuilding itself economically in the 1950s and early 1960s was something of which they were very proud.

An alternative hypothesis to the one presented by Stephens and Brynner is that, as Germany's economic success was the country's way forward from its post-war destruction, executives of successful corporations such as Grünenthal might have had a particularly strong incentive to preserve this. Beyond sheer greed, there was perhaps, in Grünenthal's reaction, a fierce impulse to reject anything which would get in the way of rebuilding the Germans' wounded national pride.

Of course, this hypothesis of ours is simply that – a hypothesis. We are merely observing that the context in which thalidomide was born might have influenced the behavior of the parties involved. In no way are we saying that Mückter's attitude was excusable.

Certainly, Mückter must have been terrified at the consequences of Contergan being withdrawn. He himself had a percentage of thalidomide's profits and was earning – according to one estimate – about 30,000 Deutschmarks per month, an enormous sum by the standards of anyone in post-war Germany.

The following quotation is the translation of a paragraph contained in a letter written in German by Carl A. Bunde, director of medical research at the Wm. S. Merrell Company. The letter was dated 15 November 1961, only fifteen days before thalidomide was withdrawn from the British market, but still before the scandal broke.

It seems that each time an article appears abroad (i.e., outside the United States) with adverse remarks about thalidomide, the Food and Drug

Administration uses this excuse to delay our new drug application even more. [author's translation]

This is a compelling illustration of how unreasonable the drug companies' priorities were at the time. Ignoring the possibility that these adverse articles might be appearing for a reason – say, the drug being unsafe – they focused on the financial inconvenience of their new drug application being delayed. One would expect the director of medical research at a major pharmaceutical company to understand why the FDA would take such articles into careful consideration before making a new drug available to the entire population of the United States.

On 25 November 1961, Mückter still refused to withdraw the drug from the market, but he did agree to issue a company letter warning of possible dangers.

However, the following day *Welt am Sonntag*, a major West German newspaper, published an article breaking the news about Lenz's findings and quoting what it considered to be the most important passage of his letter: 'that every month's delay in clarification meant that fifty to one hundred horribly mutilated children would be born'.

This news story, not surprisingly, had enormous implications for the whole country, and especially for pregnant mothers who had taken Contergan. After reading the headline and the report, Mückter reluctantly agreed to withdraw thalidomide – but only from the German market. However, Grünenthal notified licensees of the drug in other countries – including Distillers – of its decision. When doing so, Grünenthal downplayed this withdrawal as merely stemming from the 'sensationalism of the *Welt am Sonntag* story'. In spite of this, within a few days, newspapers, radio and television across Germany were alerting women not to take the drug under any circumstances.

The nightmare was now close to an end, thank goodness, though not for the many thousands of victims of thalidomide worldwide and their parents and other relatives.

On 30 November 1961, thalidomide was finally withdrawn globally by Grünenthal. However, this did not mean that every tablet of this appalling drug – appalling if you were a pregnant mother or a fetus, anyway – on pharmacy shelves and in patients' medicine cabinets around the world were suddenly thrown into the trash. If only that had been the case!

Once the demon that was thalidomide had been allowed to infest Germany's medical system, it was difficult to get this demon back into the box. A similar problem arose around the world in other countries where thalidomide had been approved.

For example, a report in the Brazilian magazine *Ocruziero* on 6 September 1962, reported that even though thalidomide was not on sale in Brazil, about fifty infants had been born in the country with phocomelia. The reporter visited a pharmacy, purchased a drug containing thalidomide and discovered that other drugs containing thalidomide were manufactured in São Paolo, then distributed all over Brazil. The Brazilian health authorities then started an investigation and found that thalidomide was sold under five different names, all unauthorized uses of the drug in a country where the health regulations were nowhere near as strong as in the United States. Fortunately, once the truth was out, a nationwide campaign was launched to take any thalidomide-containing drugs off the market. During a ten-day-long search, health authorities throughout Brazil confiscated almost two and a half million pills, forty-six thousand bottles containing thalidomide, and 96,000 kilograms of the pure substance in the pharmacies and pharmaceutical firms of São Paolo. This was all during the summer of 1962.

In Italy, thalidomide was sold under ten different trade names. In spite of an outbreak of phocomelia in Turin in June 1962, some of these products were not withdrawn in Italy until September 1962. In Argentina, thalidomide-containing drugs were not taken off the market until March 1962.

In Japan, thalidomide had first been made available under the brand names of Isomin and Pro-Ban M by the Dainippon Pharmaceutical

Company on 20 January 1958 – some two months later than Contergan. Subsequently thalidomide and compound substances containing it were produced by fourteen firms under fifteen trade names and sold without prescription. Dainippon and its products held more than 90 per cent of the Japanese market before the withdrawal of the drug.

On 17 May 1962, in view of reports they'd received from Europe associating it with congenital malformations, five of the fourteen Japanese firms supplying thalidomide to Japanese markets voluntarily decided to stop producing and selling the drug. News about thalidomide-affected babies in Europe had appeared frequently in medical journals and in newspapers in Japan, but the name 'thalidomide' was almost exclusively used, not the more familiar 'Isomin'. As a result, few doctors were aware of the connection.

On 13 September 1962, these five firms finally said that they would withdraw thalidomide-containing drugs from the market, and by January 1963, more than a year after Grünenthal had withdrawn Contergan, thalidomide was withdrawn by all Japanese firms that had supplied it. Unquestionably in Japan, hundreds of malformed babies were born as a result of pregnant mothers taking thalidomide even *after* Lenz, McBride, and others had revealed the teratogenic effects of the drug.

Lenz wrote a paper for a German medical journal describing 161 cases of malformation where Contergan had been taken by the mother. He also wrote a letter in *The Lancet* endorsing McBride's letter. The text of this is as follows:

Letter to the editor, *The Lancet*, published on January 6, 1962
THALIDOMIDE AND CONGENITAL ABNORMALITIES
SIR, – Dr McBride (Dec. 16) describes congenital abnormalities in babies delivered of women who have taken thalidomide. I have seen fifty-two malformed infants whose mothers had taken 'Contergan' in early pregnancy, and I understand that Contergan is a synonym of thalidomide, others being 'Distaval', 'Softenon', 'Neurosedyn', 'Isomin', 'Kedavon', 'Telargan', and 'Sedalis'.

Since I discussed the possible etiological role of Contergan in human malformations at a conference on November 18, 1961, I have received letters from many places in the German Federal Republic, as well as from Belgium, England, and Sweden, reporting 115 additional cases in which this drug was thought to be the cause.

Though these malformations are variable, they are of a rather specific nature. It is usually possible to infer from the type of the abnormalities alone whether Contergan has been taken. Typical of a Contergan history are defects of the arms (amelia, atypical phocomelia with absence of the thumbs and sometimes of other fingers as well, aplasia of the radius, defects of the long bones of the legs, especially the femora and tibiae, absence of the auricles, hemangiomata of the nose and the upper lip [wine-spot variety], atresia of the esophagus, the duodenum, or the anus, cardiac anomalies, and aplasia of the gallbladder and of the appendix).

Judging from case histories of more than three hundred women who have borne normal infants, and of whom none had taken Contergan between the fourth and eighth week after conception, the risk to a fetus of a mother taking Contergan during this period may be definitely higher than 20 percent.

I venture the estimate that at least two thousand, possibly more than three thousand, 'Contergan' babies have been born in Western Germany since 1959.

W. Lenz

Universitäts-Kinderklinik,

Hamburg-Eppendorf, Germany

Lenz also published a paper that specifically explained the relationship between a baby's gestation and the likelihood and nature of thalidomide damage. He said that women who took even just one tablet of thalidomide between the twentieth and thirty-sixth day of conception (the thirty-fourth and fiftieth day after the start of their last menstrual cycle) were at risk of delivering malformed infants.

Astonishingly and appallingly, Grünenthal, even after thalidomide had been withdrawn, launched a barrage of personal attacks on Lenz based on a quotation from the great German poet Goethe:

> Idiots and clever people are both equally harmless. Those halfwits and half-educated people who always recognize only half-truths alone are dangerous.

Literary-minded Chemie Grünenthal executives might have done well to apply another quotation from Goethe (from his poem 'Proverbial') to themselves:

> Just do the right thing in your affairs;
> The rest will take care of itself.

But exhorting Chemie Grünenthal to do that was a lost cause. Its executives even slandered Lenz's family, describing his father as a 'famous and popular geneticist in Nazi times', since he had 'proven the validity of the master race concept on genetic grounds'.

The Lancet printed McBride's letter, and he became a popular hero in Australia. He was named Australia's Man of the Year for 1962 and, in 1969, Queen Elizabeth made him a commander of the British Empire.

In her recollections, Frankie acknowledges that, when investigating the nature of thalidomide, she and her colleagues were handicapped by remoteness from Europe. Because of this, it took longer than they would have liked to understand what was going on there. As she says:

> Today we would just fly over to Europe and investigate this matter [the thalidomide situation] ourselves. This is one of the great benefits of the improvements in the law and the greater stress on safety and so on: we've become much more active in pursuing these clues and settling matters ourselves, not necessarily depending on second- or third-hand information. We have become much more closely allied, as it were, with food and drug establishments in other countries, with exchange of information. There are

other countries which have adopted regulatory systems, and we do have a fair exchange of information with those countries.

Frankie continues:

In November 1961 Merrell indicated to us that they would not do any further testing on the drug until they got more precise information. Merrell then sent out warning letters to doctors in the United States on December 5, 1961. This first letter only went to a rather limited number of investigators – those whose names had been submitted in the NDA, for example. So the thirty or forty investigators who were named in the new drug application were contacted, and we assumed that these were all the people that had the drug.

Frankie also notes in her memoir:

On March 8, 1962, the formal withdrawal of the application was submitted. There is nothing that would lead me to think we had requested the withdrawal. I think Merrell withdrew it of their own accord when they were finally convinced that there really was a problem relating to the drug. Until that time they were hopeful that it was not so.

You may wonder why it took Merrell five months to formally withdraw the application. But, remember, since thalidomide was never permitted to be marketed in the United States, there was no urgency to stop the application process. Once Merrell had communicated to the FDA that the drug was clearly suspect, there was no longer any danger of thalidomide being approved for distribution in the United States, whether the NDA was withdrawn or not. As Frankie reflects:

It may seem that there was a rather long period between November (1961) and March (1962) but, for any adverse reaction report like this, there is always a period of doubt where one is not sure that there is real correlation. Except for a rather small note, there were no published articles on the problems of deformities for example until about February 1962. We were aware that this drug was in the investigational stage but we felt that it was well under control by the sponsors. In other words, we believed that they had informed their investigators and had warned them.

Frankie, dignified in victory as in so many other areas of her life and professional practice, did not exult over what had happened but simply regarded it as the conclusion of a procedure that had involved Merrell applying for permission to market the drug. As far as Frankie was concerned, the matter was at an end, although she no doubt would have preferred that children around the world had not been born malformed.

Frankie tended to operate in a calm and thoughtful way. She once remarked, for example:

It has been said that I was told by [officials in the FDA], 'If you can't stand the heat, get out of the kitchen!' I cannot say I remember that.

If any of Frankie's colleagues did say this, then at the time of the thalidomide application perhaps there was a sense at the FDA that drug companies had some kind of right to put pressure on officials. Frankie admits as much in her own memoir when she explains that although there was some pressure, she thought it was 'understandable for the company to get their drugs approved'.

Frankie always seemed curiously benign about how Merrell had treated her. It's difficult not to feel that she was kinder than it deserved. The company's attitude in the context of its thalidomide application would have made anyone furious, wouldn't it?

Righteous anger is one of the traits we associate with typical heroes. Something from the baser regions of human nature (be it greed, selfishness, negligence or outright cruelty) sparks a tragedy – that's how the story starts. Infuriated by the resulting suffering, the hero sets out to destroy the cause: an enemy that is now considered to be entirely evil, and for whom no mercy shall be shown.

Such an emphasis has been placed on this kind of heroism that Frankie's measured reaction barely makes sense to us. How was she so calm in the face of Merrell's behavior? After she learned what terrible damage their greed could have caused, how did she find it in herself not to slander them for their negligence?

What at first glance seems an overly tempered reaction is actually evidence of a rare strand of strength. Anger and passion are easy to indulge. The true challenge is never to get contaminated by the lower instincts of the Merrells of this world, but instead to remain calm, rational and kind.

Frankie's heroism partly stemmed from her impressive ability not to take Merrell's attitude personally. She could have let herself be darkened by the way she was being treated. When she told the story years later in her memoir, she could have used her moral high ground to paint a wholly unforgiving picture of the company. She could have basked victoriously in the somber pleasure we tend to draw from uttering the delightful words: 'I told you so'.

But she didn't. During the whole thalidomide saga, she remained focused on one essential thing: the facts of the case. Personal feelings about the company or the drug had no place in her work. Because of her unaltered professionalism, her judgment remained clear. What could Merrell have done against her, when her objections to the thalidomide application were all, without fail, based on hard evidence – not on passions or grudges? In contrast, Dr Murray's outbursts of emotion didn't stand a chance. It is likely that this helped Frankie to retain the trust of her superiors at the FDA on the occasions when Merrell attempted to go over her head.

Frankie's recollection of the events is solely based on facts, as was her work on the thalidomide application. As any worthy scientist, she built an analysis which included the perspective and situation of all parties involved, rather than just her own. Her purpose was not to pass judgement, but simply to explain what had happened: what Merrell did, what it didn't do, and what the results were.

This outstanding ability for stoicism and objectivity, though hugely underrated, is among the most impressive qualities a hero can possess.

That said, Frankie certainly didn't consider herself a heroine. The world, however, soon felt very differently.

Thirteen

THE WORLD STARTS TO RECOGNIZE A HEROINE

It was an article in the Sunday edition of *The Washington Post* on 15 July 1962, by a science journalist named Morton Mintz that started Frankie's much-deserved elevation to the status of a celebrity heroine.

HEROINE OF FDA KEEPS BAD DRUG OFF MARKET
By Morton Mintz, Staff Reporter

This is the story of how the skepticism and stubbornness of a government physician prevented what could have been an appalling American tragedy, the birth of hundreds or indeed thousands of armless and legless children.

The story of Dr Frances Oldham Kelsey, a Food and Drug Administration medical officer, is not one of inspired prophesies nor of dramatic research breakthroughs.

She saw her duty in sternly simple terms, and she carried it out, living the while with insinuations that she was a bureaucratic nitpicker, unreasonable – even, she said, stupid. That such attributes could have been ascribed to her is, by her own acknowledgement, not surprising, considering all of the circumstances.

What she did was refuse to be hurried into approving an application for marketing a new drug. She regarded its safety as unproved, despite considerable data arguing that it was ultra safe.

It was not until last April, [eight] months after the application was filed with the FDA, that the terrible effects of the drug abroad were widely reported in this country. What remains to be told is how and why Dr Kelsey blocked the introduction of the drug before those effects were suspected by anyone.

Dr Kelsey invoked her high standards and her belief that the drug was 'peculiar' against these facts:

The drug had come into widespread use in other countries. In West Germany, where it was used primarily as a sedative, huge quantities of it were sold over the counter before it was put on a prescription basis. It gave a prompt, deep, natural sleep that was not followed by a hangover. It was cheap. It failed to kill even the would-be suicides who swallowed massive doses.

And there were reports on experiments with animals. Only a few weeks ago the American licensee told of giving the drug to rats in doses of six to sixty times greater than the comparable human dosage. Of 1510 offspring, none was delivered with 'evidence of malformation'.

In a separate study, one rat did deliver a malformed offspring, but the dosage had been 120 times the usual one. Rabbits that were injected with six times the comparable human dose also were reported to have produced no malformed births.

Recently, the FDA publicly decried the 'excessive contacts' made by pharmaceutical manufacturers who are anxious to speed the agency's handling of new drug applications.

Many Requests

So it was not at all surprising that dozens of contacts were made with Dr Kelsey by representatives of the American licensee for thalidomide, the chemical name for the sedative. They had what they strongly believed was a clear and overwhelming case – but Dr Kelsey delayed, and delayed, and delayed.

They visited her drably furnished, bare-floor office in an eyesore temp on Jefferson Dr., SW. They phoned. They submitted a flow of reports and studies. It was apparent that substantial investments and substantial profits were at stake. And all of this was routine.

The application had come to Dr Kelsey – simply because it was her turn to take the next one in September, 1960.

The European data left her 'very unimpressed'. In an interview, she said she had 'lived through cycles before' in which a drug was acclaimed for a year or two – until harmful side effects became known.

And, she said she could not help regarding thalidomide as a 'peculiar drug'. It troubled her that its effects on experimental animals were not the same as on humans – it did not make them sleepy.

Same Questions

Could there be danger in those few people whose systems might absorb it? Could there be a harmful effect on the unborn child whose mother took it? (In other countries obstetricians were innocently prescribing it as an anti-emetic for pregnant women.)

Dr Kelsey regarded the manufacturer's evidence of thalidomide's safety as 'incomplete in many respects'. The drug was not, after all, intended for grave diseases, or for the relief of intolerable suffering, but primarily for sleeplessness, for which many drugs of known safety were already on the market.

All of this being so, she saw no need either to hurry or to be satisfied with the approach that, nine chances out of ten, it's safe. She was determined to be certain that thalidomide was safe ten times out of ten, and she was prepared to wait forever for proof that it was.

When the sixty-day deadline for action on the application came around, Dr Kelsey wrote the manufacturer that the proof of safety was inadequate. Perhaps with an understandable feeling of frustration the manufacturer produced new research data, new reasons for action. Each time a new sixty-day deadline drew near, out went another letter: insufficient proof of safety.

Upheld by Superiors

Dr Kelsey's tenacity – or unreasonableness, depending upon one's viewpoint – was upheld by her superiors, all the way.

Although she takes her work seriously indeed, her contacts with applicants are, in her words, 'usually amiable. We see their point, and they see ours. But the responsibility for releasing a drug is ours, not theirs'. And that is the responsibility she would not forget.

In February, 1961, she chanced to read, in a British medical journal, a letter from a British doctor questioning whether certain instances of peripheral neuritis – a tingling numbness in the feet and the fingers that is sometimes irreversible – might not be due to intake of thalidomide. To her this was a danger signal.

She called the letter to the attention of the applicant. His investigators reported that the incidence was apparently negligible, one case among 300,000 adult users. Six months later, Dr Kelsey said, the incidence among adults who took thalidomide regularly for months at a time was found to be one in 250.

But neither she nor the applicant yet had the slightest inkling that the drug could be responsible for the birth of malformed babies. That awful circumstantial evidence became known to the applicant – in a cablegram from Europe – on November 29, 1961.

Application Withdrawn

He reported it to Dr Kelsey early the next day. Although this was followed by a formal withdrawal of the application, as late as last month the applicant described the birth abnormalities as 'alleged effects' of thalidomide.

The story begins in 1954, six years before Dr Kelsey, a pharmacologist as well as a physician, went to work in the FDA's Bureau of Medicine. She and her husband, F. Ellis Kelsey, a pharmacologist who is now a special assistant to the Surgeon General of the Public Health Service, came from the faculty of the University of South Dakota School of Medicine.

For the account that follows, the primary sources were Dr Kelsey and reports by Dr Helen B. Taussig to a medical meeting in April and in the June 30 issue of *The Journal of the American Medical Association.*

Morton Mintz's article continues with background information on thalidomide, much of which has been covered already in this book. He refers to Dr Helen Taussig and her enthusiasm for strengthening the 1939 Food and Drug Act 'to provide greater assurance that new drugs would not harm unborn children'.

Mintz then concludes his article as follows:

But to Assistant FDA Commissioner Winton B. Rankin, the significant thing about the law is that it gave Dr Kelsey the weapon she needed to block the marketing of thalidomide in the United States.

'The American public', he said, 'owes her a vote of thanks'.

The forty-seven-year-old Dr Kelsey lives at 5811 Brookside Dr, Chevy Chase, with her husband and daughters, Susan, fifteen, and Christine, twelve.

She is grateful for the praise – but recognizes that, had thalidomide proved to be as safe as the applicant believed, 'I would have been considered unreasonable'.

She intends to go on 'playing for that tenth chance in ten' to assure safety in new drugs 'to the best of my ability'. For twenty years she taught pharmacology. She knows the dangers, and she has not the slightest intention of forgetting them.

Morton Mintz, who was born on 26 January 1922, was interviewed on 27 April 2007, by Professor Charles Lewis, executive editor of the Investigative Reporting Workshop, about the impact Frankie's story and the peril of thalidomide made on him. We've already quoted from this interview at the beginning of this book, but here is a transcription of the full interview, used by kind permission of the Investigative Reporting Workshop.

CL: You have written that it changed your life profoundly, that story. Can you describe – just go into it ...

MM: Thalidomide, as you know, was a drug that caused ... women who took it in the first trimester for the nausea of pregnancy ... to give birth to babies without arms or without legs or without any limbs at all, and it was invented in Germany under the name Contergan, as I remember. And there was a drug company based in Cincinnati that wanted to market it here. I knew nothing about drugs or the FDA or anything else, and in the interview I was just absolutely shocked to hear that this drug company had applied the pressures on Dr Kelsey. I mean, it was outrageous. I wrote the story. It appeared the morning after we left on vacation on July 15, 1962, and it set off a huge storm. I think she had done her duty in keeping this drug off the market, and it was transformational in the sense that it was the first personal awakening that really mattered as to what corporate conduct can be, how bad it can be, how criminal it can be in some cases. That's what it was, I think, more than anything else.

CL: I'm sorry to digress about it. Didn't you end up getting a Nieman fellowship around this matter?

MM: That was I guess clearly a key factor, maybe *the* key factor in my getting a Nieman fellowship to Harvard, which began in the fall of 1962, and I had an interview with one of the then-sponsors of the program after we arrived – it was Arthur Schlessinger Senior, professor of history, and he told me that that was a big factor.

CL: Was it difficult for that ... well, you had an editor who was interested also it sounds like in getting it published. It was not an issue, the publishing.

MM: Oh, no, it ran on page one.

CL: And just to close the loop on what happened with thalidomide. Wasn't thalidomide banned?

MM: It was never approved for the market even though thousands of 'experimental' doses had been distributed in the United States. It was just horrifying.

Charles Lewis writes about Morton Mintz in his 2014 book *935 Lies: The Future of Truth and the Decline of America's Moral Integrity*

His story epitomizes many of the trials facing anyone who dedicates his life to the pursuit of truth in a world where powerful interests prefer secrecy and deception.

In 1962, Mintz wrote a remarkable front-page story for the *Post* about Dr Frances Oldham Kelsey, a Food and Drug Administration (FDA) official who had resisted intense pressure from the pharmaceutical industry to approve the sedative thalidomide (trade name Kevadon) for sale to pregnant women suffering from morning sickness. Of course, thalidomide was later found to cause severe deformities in the children of pregnant mothers who used it, including missing arms or legs. His incisive journalism inflamed and emboldened Congress to enact legislation giving the FDA greater authority to require that drug companies scientifically test and prove that their products are safe.

Within weeks of Mintz's story, President John F. Kennedy specifically commended Frankie by name during a nationally televised press conference, and days after that he presented her with the President's Award for Distinguished Federal Civilian Service. Soon after, Congress unanimously passed and signed into law tougher federal controls regulating the safety and effectiveness of pharmaceutical drugs. Frankie's honor was announced in a press release dated Friday, 3 August 1962, from the Department of Health, Education, and Welfare.

President Kennedy presented Frankie with her medal on Tuesday, 7 August 1962. Once the significance of her contribution was understood by the US government, it didn't waste any time. There is a grainy YouTube video, just over a minute long, showing Frankie on her way to the ceremony in an elegant black outfit. At one point, she pauses outside the White House for photographs with her elder daughter Susan, as tall as Frankie, on her left, and Christine on her right, with a hairband in her hair. The ceremony took place on the lawn of the White House. After shaking hands with Frankie, President Kennedy placed the medal around her neck, taking a few moments to ensure it was arranged neatly at the back. It was one of the finest moments in the history of the United States. Today, President Kennedy is perhaps most remembered for being assassinated on 22 November the following year. Let's remember that he was elected because millions believed he could bring the promise of a new wave of youthful idealism and a sense of moral purpose to the business of government. On that bright August day in 1962, handing Frankie her richly deserved honor, that promise was abundantly fulfilled.

Six days earlier, during a remarkable press conference, President Kennedy had praised Frankie and outlined the steps that were being taken to ensure that thalidomide was no longer a threat in the United States. What follows is from the president's press conference from the new State Department auditorium in Washington, D.C., 1 August 1962.

JFK: Afternoon, I have several announcements. Recent events in this country and abroad concerning the effects of a new sedative called thalidomide emphasize again the urgency of providing additional protection to American consumers from harmful or worthless drug products.

The United States has the best and most effective food and drug law of any country in the world, and the alert work of our Food and Drug Administration, and particularly Dr Frances Kelsey, prevented this particular drug from being distributed commercially in this country. Nevertheless, the drug was given to many patients on an investigational basis. We are reviewing what steps can be taken administratively to make this stage in the future less dangerous.

We have recommended a 25-percent increase in the Food and Drug Administration staff, the largest single increase in the agency's history, and the full amount was voted today by the conferees of the Congress, and it is clear that to prevent even more serious disasters occurring in this country in the future, additional legislative safeguards are necessary. The bill reported by the Senate Judiciary Committee on July 19th, while embodying many of the recommendations contained in the message of March this year, does not go far enough, as Senator Kefauver and others have pointed out in their supplementary review on the committee report.

I hope the members of Congress will adopt those more careful provisions contained in the administration bill introduced by Congressman Aaron Harris of Arkansas in the House. The Administration Bill, for example, unlike the Senate Judiciary Bill, will allow for immediate removal from the market of a new drug where there is an immediate hazard to public health which cannot be done now and contains with it many other very essential safeguards which I hope the Congress will act on this year.

Secondly, we are completing a careful review of the technical problems associated with an effective test ban treaty.

This review was stimulated by important new technical assessments. These assessments give promise that we can work towards an internationally supervised system of detection and verification for underground testing which will be simpler and more economical than the system which was contained in the treaty which we tabled in Geneva in April 1961.

I must emphasize that these new assessments do not affect the requirement that any system must include provision for on-site inspection of unidentified underground events. It may be that we shall not need as many as we have needed in the past, but we find no justification for the Soviet claim that a test ban treaty can be effective without on-site inspection.

We have been conducting a most careful and intensive review of our whole position, with the object of bringing it squarely in line with the technical realities. I must express the hope that the Soviet government too will reexamine its position on this matter of inspection. In the past it has accepted the principle, and if it would return to this earlier position, we for our part will be able to engage in an attempt to reach agreement on the number of on-site inspections which is essential. Ambassador Arthur

Dean has been participating in these deliberations and will be returning to Geneva promptly. He will be prepared for intensive technical discussions of these problems.

And finally I want to express my very strong hope that the House of Representatives will give approval to the UN bond proposal. The UN is engaged at this very time in two very important negotiations, one involving the Congo, the other involving the future of West Africa, and it is daily proving its effectiveness and maintaining the peace and the stability of much of the world. This would be a most unfortunate time if we withdrew our support from it, and I'm hopeful that the House will follow the Senate's example and give us the power to participate in this UN bond program which I believe to be essential to its survival, just as I believe that the survival of the United Nations is essential for the peace of the world.

Question: Mr. President, in connection with your opening statement about this period of anguish over the use of this drug with women asking for abortions, there apparently has been some difficulty with people running down all the remaining stocks of thalidomide still in this country. Is there anything short of what you told us, or is there anything additional that the government can do without legislation, to run down these remaining supplies of this drug and take it into custody?

JFK: The Food and Drug Administration have had nearly two hundred people working on this. Every doctor, every hospital, every nurse has been notified. Every woman in this country I think must be aware that it is most important that they check their medicine cabinet, that they do not take this drug, that they turn it in. Every citizen of course should be aware of the hazards, and I'm sure they are. Now what we have to concern ourselves about is, first, the appreciation to Dr Kelsey, who spared us this terrible human tragedy which has been visited on families in Germany, and to provide both administrative and legislative safeguards to lessen the chance of such action coming in this country again. Also I think to see if we can assist

... other countries in providing effective safeguards for their own citizens, because the interrelationship between them and us is very intimate.

After Frankie received her medal, her elevation to the status of national hero soon gained more and more momentum. There was an ad called 'Drug Detective' sponsored by the FDA that focused on Frankie's work in preventing the distribution of thalidomide. This advertisement was designed and sponsored by the Federal Civil Service and featured the slogan 'Four Score Years of Service to America'.

More plaudits were given to Frankie during the rest of 1962 and beyond. Another example is an article appearing in the *Catholic Standard* on Friday, 10 August 1962, by Mary Tinley Daly, which makes the following comment about Frankie:

All heroines are not out battling fire, flood, and disaster. Some are in homes, offices, classrooms, laboratories.

Such a heroine is Dr Frances O. Kelsey, medical officer with the US Food and Drug Administration, who Tuesday was presented with the President's Award for Distinguished Federal Civilian Service by President Kennedy at a ceremony at the White House.

'Many people must be nominated for this award', Dr Kelsey shrugged when interviewed in her comfortable suburban home. 'We were pleased, of course ['We' being her, her husband, and her two daughters], but I only did what I thought was right'.

The slender Dr Kelsey, who was praised by President Kennedy at his press conference last week, is a serenely calm woman with sparkling brown eyes who looks far younger than her forty-seven years. Short brown hair is brushed back with the casual sophistication of a thoroughbred. Her manner is pleasant but unhurried, and one senses that her responsibilities are not taken lightly.

This has been proven. You will recall reading that she kept off the American market a drug believed to be responsible for malformation of infants. Thousands of babies, in other countries, whose mothers took the sleeping pill in early pregnancy, were born without arms or legs, with seal-like 'flippers' attached to shoulder or hip, and with other malformations.

Pharmacologist and mother, as well as physician, Dr Kelsey asked this reporter about the use of drugs not thoroughly tested and declared safe. The drug she stopped is the now widely publicized thalidomide, marketed in other countries under various trade names.

Asked how she did such a marvelous tragedy-preventing job in this country, Dr Kelsey said, 'I found something peculiar about it, in spite of all the claims for its excellence'.

Mary Daly points out that Frankie first found something 'peculiar' about thalidomide in September 1960, which is three months before the news broke that the drug caused infant deformities.

Mary Daly continues:

Proponents of the drug found something decidedly 'peculiar' about Dr Kelsey. She was an obstructionist, to their way of thinking, a bureaucrat who was acting unreasonably in the light of overwhelming evidence.

On 16 July 1962, Mrs Christina B. Martan sent the following letter to Frankie.

Dear Dr Kelsey,

Thank you – not for being right, but for having the courage to stick by your convictions. For caring about what happens to other people's babies.

...

The applicants' urgency to sell their product without concern for the result is the most revolting thing, but not surprising is the fact that it has happened before, in some cases without even an apparent good reason for the use of the product.

Perhaps this story will cause some people to have a little more care in the use of new drugs, unless in extreme necessity.

Think I'll stick to aspirins.

Yours most sincerely,

Mrs Christina B. Martan

Mrs Martan was only too right; Merrell's behavior was 'revolting', right up to the time of its shamefaced withdrawal of the thalidomide NDA.

On 21 July 1962, the following letter was published in *The Lancet*. The author was Mr. Tadashi Kajii from the Department of Pediatrics, Hokkaido University Hospital, Sapporo, Hokkaido, Japan. It is titled 'Thalidomide and Congenital Deformities':

Sir. Having read recent contributions in your columns, a no doubt retrospective study for infants born in seven major hospitals of Sapporo, Japan, I found several cases of severe phocomelia born within a period of just over ten months, the first on August 8, 1961. The annual delivery rate for this hospital group averages six thousand. I can find no record of any previous local case of this condition, certainly none in the three years preceding my first case.

In five of these seven cases, the mothers were definitely on thalidomide during the early weeks of pregnancy. One of these babies showed how small a dose of thalidomide is sufficient to produce a typical deformity. The mother took thirty milligrams of thalidomide at night for nine days after a menstrual period had been overdue for a week. This dose is a little less than that of a case recorded by Mr. Stabler. The baby died at seven days and had severe phocomelia with microphthalmia, interventricular septal defect, absent gall bladder, cryptorchidism, hydronephrosis, and absent horizontal fissure in the right lung. Another two cases in this series had coccygeal fovia in addition to limb deformity.

I estimate that approximately seven hundred babies with phocomelia had been born in Japan since 1961. Thalidomide was withdrawn from the market of this country in May 1962.

Less than four months later, on 15 October 1962, a short article appeared in the United States journal *Modern Medicine*. The headline was 'Safety and Skepticism: Thalidomide'.

> Between Capitol Hill and the Washington Monument is a plain two-story building that has been 'temporary' since The Second World War. The first floor is occupied by the Medical Museum of the Armed Forces Institute of Pathology. Until the thalidomide episode, few knew or cared that the second floor was the home of the New Drugs Division, the Bureau of Medicine, United States Food [and Drug] Administration. Then the spotlight fell on an unusual group of physicians who have responsibility for giving the go-ahead to the marketing of new drugs.
>
> Performing no experiments, examining no patients, working in drab offices piled with documents, the twelve full-time medical officers of the Division are paid $13,510 or so annually to be skeptics. 'We're not infallible', says one medical officer, a former pharmacology professor and one-time private practitioner in South Dakota. She is Dr Frances Oldham Kelsey, who won a presidential award for her part in keeping thalidomide off the US prescription market. Disclaiming sole credit, she says her colleagues shared in the decision ...

Early in 1963 the FDA presented evidence that Merrell had abused its 'investigational use' privilege by engaging in commercialism when it distributed thalidomide to doctors for investigative use, and that the drug was misbranded by false assertions regarding its safety. However, the FDA's case did not apparently greatly impress the Justice Department. One staff member reported that he spoke to the Justice Department lawyers until he was 'blue in the face', but he was certain the case would not be brought.

On 21 September 1964, the FDA received confirmation from the officials. A letter from the Justice Department stated in part that the Department had concluded the criminal prosecution was neither warranted nor desirable. The letter continued:

This case ... does not seem sufficiently strong or clear to be the subject of a criminal prosecution. Some 'promotional' aspects of the Merrell company's distribution of Kevadon no doubt have questionable overtones. However it seems the regulations or instructions then in force did not specifically proscribe such practices. Considering the regulations as a whole, without the benefit of hindsight, it seems difficult to maintain that Merrell deliberately or culpably misconstrued them in this matter. Rather Merrell seems to have acted in good faith and to have been innocent of intent to violate the regulations.

Subsequently the FDA strongly urged the Justice Department to reconsider its decision, because as one staff member put it, 'We are merely going through the motions so that the records show we didn't take a back seat'.

Efforts by the FDA to bring a criminal case against Merrell failed, but the avenue of civil action by private citizens was still very much open. Up to 1973 at least thirteen claims had been brought against Merrell in the United States (additional suits were brought by Canadians in that country). At that time some of the cases had been settled out of court. These cases related to the mercifully small number of thalidomide-affected babies born in the United States – the results of the drug being supplied to pregnant women by their doctors for investigational purposes.

The Justice Department's refusal to prosecute the case against Merrell did at least point out the need for a tighter restriction of the FDA's regulations about control of drugs at the investigational level. The days when drug companies could simply supply doctors with any drug, no matter how potentially toxic, for investigational purposes were coming to an end. New regulations went into effect on 7 February 1963. These regulations said that a company planning to undertake a clinical investigation had to tell the FDA of its plans, including information concerning the pre-clinical studies, as well as the number of qualifications of the investigators and what the precise nature of the study was. The company then had to monitor the progress of the studies and report its findings to the FDA at specified periods. Moreover, all investigators – that is, the doctors involved – had to sign a statement affirming that they understood the conditions applying to the use of investigational drugs, which included adequate records of receipt and names of people to whom the drug was given. Best of all, perhaps, the FDA was given the power to terminate the investigation on numerous grounds including evidence that the drug was being commercialized, substantial evidence that the drug was unsafe, or evidence that the company sponsoring the program failed to submit progress reports.

The US Kefauver Harris Amendment, or 'Drug Efficacy Amendment', is a 1962 amendment to the Federal Food, Drug, and Cosmetic Act. It introduced a requirement for drug manufacturers to provide proof of the effectiveness and safety of their drugs before approval, required drug advertising to disclose accurate information about side effects, and stopped cheap generic drugs being marketed as expensive drugs under new trade names as new 'breakthrough' medications.

The amendment was a response to the thalidomide scandal. It was brought before Congress by US Senator Estes Kefauver, of Tennessee, and US Representative Oren Harris, of Arkansas.

The new legislation introduced by Senator Kefauver in the United States was radical in several respects. First of all, the provision in the old law that automatically allowed a drug to go on the market was removed completely. Under the new law, the FDA had to give its positive consent before any drug could go onto the market. This eliminated the clumsy need – which prevailed when Frankie was investigating thalidomide – for the FDA to declare an NDA as incomplete and demand its resubmission after sixty days. In addition, the FDA was given the power to withdraw any drug if new information indicated that it was an imminent hazard to the public health.

To the old requirement that a manufacturer had to prove to the FDA that a drug was safe, the new law added the requirement that the manufacturer had to prove the drug was also efficacious in treatment of the ailments for which it was intended. Drug companies were required by the new law to notify the FDA immediately of any reports of adverse effects associated with the drug, both during the clinical phase and after marketing. Perhaps most significant of all, according to many commentators, was that an amendment in the law, prompted from the floor by Senators Jacob Javits and John A. Carroll which stipulated that patients, except under certain conditions, had to be informed if they were being given an experimental drug.

The new law was signed by President John F. Kennedy on 10 October 1962.

Senator Kefauver was a charming, warm-hearted, right-minded man who liked people (on 18 March 1951, he made a memorable and entertaining appearance on the popular TV show *What's My Line?*) and was quite indignant about the US's extremely narrow escape from thalidomide.

If history had worked out a little differently, Kefauver could have become president of the United States. After leading a highly publicized investigation into organized crime in the early 1950s, Kefauver twice sought his party's nomination for president. In 1956 he was chosen by the Democratic National Convention to be the running mate of presidential nominee Adlai Stevenson. Still holding his US Senate seat after the Stevenson–Kefauver ticket lost to the Eisenhower–Nixon ticket in 1956, Kefauver was named chair of the US Senate Antitrust and Monopoly Subcommittee in 1957 and remained as its chairman until his death in August 1963, at the early age of 60.

In November 1963, President Kennedy named Senator Kefauver's widow Nancy Kefauver to be the first head of the new Art in Embassies Program. This was President Kennedy's last presidential appointment before his tragic assassination in Dallas on 22 November 1963.

The federal courthouse in Nashville, Tennessee, was renamed the Estes Kefauver Federal Building and United States Courthouse in Senator Kefauver's honor.

Fourteen

THE CANADIAN EXPERIENCE OF THALIDOMIDE

William S. Merrell was, unfortunately, successful in its bid to get thalidomide authorized for distribution in Canada, though thankfully Kevadon – Merrell used the same brand name for the drug in Canada that it so ardently wished to use in the United States – was only available for a few months.

On 8 September 1960, four days before Frankie received the application for the authorization of thalidomide at the FDA, Merrell submitted data for thalidomide to the Food and Drug Directorate (FDD) in Ottawa. There was no resistance to approving the application, and on 22 November 1960, the FDD authorized the drug to be marketed.

This marketing began on 1 April 1961, an appropriate day considering that everyone involved in this enterprise was a fool. From the outset, Merrell included a warning about the dangers of peripheral neuritis with each Kevadon product. However, this warning was formulated in a misleading fashion: it stated that the symptoms of peripheral neuritis would disappear upon withdrawal of the medication. As we've seen, this was not the case at all, and peripheral neuritis caused by thalidomide could often be permanent.

There was another brand of thalidomide distributed in Canada by a firm called the Frank W. Horner Company. On 1 September 1961, it informed the Food and Drug Directorate in Ottawa of its intention to distribute the drug under the name Talimol. Because Kevadon was already approved for distribution in Canada, on 11 October 1961, Talimol was cleared for sale. There was even a third organization, Strong Cobb Arner of Canada Limited, which was manufacturing Kevadon tablets for Merrell by the end of 1961. However, the knowledge of what thalidomide could really do to unborn children broke at the end of November, so these second and third culprits in the disaster did not have much time to sell their drugs.

Not surprisingly, when the news broke, Dr C.A. Morrell of the FDD, who had approved thalidomide for distribution in Canada, was presented with a considerable quandary. Yet, by the end of February 1962 thalidomide had still not been banned in Canada. The *Toronto Star* queried this situation and asked Morrell whether there had been any cases of phocomelia, but he informed the newspaper that no cases had occurred.

This was in spite of an article published in *Time* magazine on 23 February 1962, entitled 'Sleeping Pill Nightmare', which was a short history of the thalidomide disaster, and included information about the findings of Lenz. While the article did not contain much in the way of speculation about the whole situation, Murray of Merrell wrote to Dr Morrell to declare that he was 'shocked by the sensational approach and the lack of objectivity' of the *Time* magazine article. It was astonishing that Murray could write like this when the drug had *already* been taken off the market in Germany and the United Kingdom, whereas Merrell itself had only sent out a warning letter to physicians who were testing the drug. Of course, thanks to Frankie, thalidomide was never approved for general sale in the United States.

But it was very clear that, even as late in the day as February 1962, Merrell was still trying to bolster its position. As for Morrell (it's not only that the similarity of the names is confusing here, but in their own way both Merrell and Morrell were complicit in what was happening with thalidomide), he claimed that when he spoke to the *Toronto Star* any connection between thalidomide and malformation was 'only statistical' – an outrageous thing to say in February 1962, when the link between thalidomide and malformation was unequivocally proven. Kev Donnellon, born with short arms, abnormal fingers and no legs at all, only feet, was undeniable proof of the dangers of thalidomide.

Thalidomide became available in 'sample tablet form' in Canada in late 1959 and was licensed for prescription use on 1 April 1961. Although it had been withdrawn from the West German and United Kingdom markets by 2 December 1961, thalidomide remained legally available in Canada until 2 March 1962, a full three months later. Amazingly, thalidomide was still available in some Canadian pharmacies until mid May 1962.

But the truth about what was happening was on the verge of coming out. On 27 February 1962, Dr Gordon Hewitson, a physician in Pointe Claire, Quebec, wrote to Dr Morrell:

Six weeks ago I saw an infant with the congenital abnormality of phocomelia (seal limbs).

In the first eight weeks of her pregnancy this mother took a daily tablet of thalidomide (Kevadon).

This drug, as you are well aware, has been removed from the market in Great Britain and never licensed for use in the United States.

The firm marketing the drug in Canada sent out a warning notice to doctors in December, and a follow-up notice was distributed last week. This hardly seems enough for such a hazardous drug; it should certainly be removed forthwith from further use.

On 1 March, another senior doctor wrote to Morrell:

I'm afraid that there can be little doubt with the accumulating literature on the subject, of which I know you are well aware, that there is more than a casual relationship between this drug and the occurrence of serious abnormalities in newborn infants.

In Canada the number of reports increased connecting phocomelia with thalidomide, and finally, on 2 March Morrell requested that all manufacturers of thalidomide in Canada withdraw the drug from the market. Yet, the tone of the letter that he wrote to the thalidomide manufacturers brings a sense that he made this request unwillingly:

A meeting was held at this Directorate on Wednesday, March 1, 1962, to discuss the advisability of *temporarily* withdrawing the drug thalidomide from the Canadian market [italics added].

In view of increasing demands from Canadian physicians, as well as certain other pressures, we have decided to ask you to withdraw your product Talimol from the Canadian market until such time as we can be certain of its possible association or lack of association with congenital deformities in newborn children. I regret very much having to take this course of action and can only hope for an early resolution of the problem.

Despite this request, according to *MacLean's* magazine of May 1962, thalidomide was still being sold over Canadian chemist counters six weeks later. An assiduous reporter for *MacLean's* had taken the trouble to phone seventy-seven chemists in eleven Canadian cities. Although he found that the drug was not being sold in any stores in Victoria, Vancouver, Regina, Winnipeg, Quebec City, Fredericton or Halifax (Winnipeg pharmacists were even upset by the journalist's question and told him they were refunding customers who brought back partly empty bottles), in Toronto, five out of twenty-four drugstores were still selling thalidomide; in Edmonton three out of eight were selling it; in Montreal three out of thirteen; and in the Ottawa-Hull area three out of eight. The journalist asked one Toronto pharmacist why thalidomide was still available for sale. The pharmacist answered, 'Why not? It is safe for the adult male, isn't it?' When the journalist pointed out that any medicine lying at home might be taken by a woman, he replied: 'That's not my problem. I'm not sending back the rest of the supply until people stop asking for it'. Hardly an ethical response.

The FDD in Ottawa, which had taken no measures to ensure that the withdrawal was effected, was told of the situation by the journal. Even Morrell was spurred to action by this new revelation, and he sent further instructions to the Canadian manufacturers:

> With the withdrawal of this acceptance thalidomide returned to the stages of a new drug and must not be sold except to qualify the investigators for the purpose of obtaining scientific and clinical information that could be used to support the safety of its use under conditions to be recommended by the manufacturer. Such sale does not include any sale to pharmacists.
>
> Violation of the new drug regulations, e.g., sale of this drug by a pharmacist, may result in seizure of the product and/or prosecution of the seller.

Not surprisingly, as the dilatory attitude of the FDD in Ottawa to the whole thalidomide nightmare began to become better known, there was public outrage against how the directorate under Morrell was behaving. On 30 March the *Toronto Globe and Mail* reported a session in the Canadian Parliament as saying that three months had elapsed between the issuing of a warning that the sedative might be dangerous to pregnant women and a government request that it be withdrawn from circulation.

Outside the House, health minister J. Waldo Monteith was pressed on the matter, but denied there had been any delay in obtaining withdrawal of the drug. As he put it: 'The department had to check rumors that were of a sketchy nature; little more than rumors', he said, and subsequently announced in Parliament:

> The information applied was statistical in nature in that the instances of certain malformations in the group of children born to mothers taking the

drug was somewhat higher than in the group of children from mothers not taking the drug.

This response to the thalidomide situation by the health minister of one of the leading democracies in the world is totally inexplicable, especially since on 3 February 1962, Dr Lenz, who had already sounded his warning about thalidomide, made his point even more strongly in a letter published in *The Lancet*.

Sir,

I am afraid I have not made my point sufficiently clear in my letter of January 6th. I have conclusive evidence that 'Contergan' (thalidomide) is teratogenic in man. The evidence includes:

(1) Six cases in which the mother disclosed before delivery that she had taken thalidomide in early pregnancy and in which the infant showed major malformations at birth of the same type as seen in retrospectively ascertained cases. Four of these cases are part of three unselected series of hospital births in which (a) no case was found in which the mother of a normal infant had taken thalidomide between the third and eighth weeks after conception, and (b) no case of the thalidomide type of malformations was found in which the mother had *not* taken the drug.

(2) Fifty-five cases in which the exact date of the prescription and/or intake of thalidomide is known and coincides with the time of development of the malformed organs.

(3) Five series of consecutive cases collected independently from hospitals outside Hamburg and communicated to me by gynecologists and pediatricians.

Lenz concludes his letter:

The number of cases known to me of malformations and the history of thalidomide intake during the first two months of pregnancy is increasing at present at a rate of three to ten per day.

As the Thalidomide Victims Association of Canada explains:

In 1987, the War Amputations of Canada established The Thalidomide Task Force to seek compensation for Canadian-born thalidomide victims from the government of Canada. As Canada had allowed the drug onto the Canadian market when many warnings were already available about side effects associated with thalidomide, and as Canada left the drug on the market a full three months after the majority of the world had withdrawn the drug, it was felt and argued that the government of Canada had a moral responsibility to ensure that thalidomide victims were properly compensated.

In 1991, the Ministry of National Health and Welfare (now Health Canada), through an 'Extraordinary Assistance Plan' awarded small compassionate lump-sum financial assistance grants to Canadian-born thalidomiders. These payments were quickly used by individuals to cover some of the extraordinary costs of their disabilities, and for most victims, these monies are long gone.

Fifteen

FRESH HONORS

For the rest of Frankie's life, honors came to her regularly, thick and fast, yet she never lost her sense of proportion, or her sense of humor. Never was there a greater heroine than Frankie, nor a more modest one.

As an example of Frankie's sense of humor, here is a memorandum she sent to Mr James Shipp, Chief Administrative Management Branch, from Frances O. Kelsey, MD, Chief Investigational Drug Branch. Subject: Erroneous information. Date: 22 April 1965. The text reads:

> I have learned ... in the past two days that at least two persons have tried to contact me by telephone but in each case have been told by the FDA operator that I no longer work for the Food and Drug Administration.
>
> If I have been fired will you please give me formal notification of this, or if the operator is in error, will you please see that this is rectified.

The handwritten reply from Mr Shipp said:

Dr Kelsey: I have checked this out with GSA, HEW, and [illegible] operators. Naturally, all plead ignorance. They all have a record of your location and telephone extension. I don't think this will come up again. Signed, J. Shipp.

This at a time when Frankie was not only the chief of the Investigational Drug Branch of the FDA, but also the world-famous savior of America who had been honored by President Kennedy.

The following is from a newspaper article in *The Washington Post* dated Thursday, 9 March 1967:

This is Women's Week in the federal service. President Johnson met Tuesday with the six winners of the coveted Federal Women's Award, and the winners were further honored at a stacked-up Hilton dinner that evening.

Mr. Johnson was given a report yesterday, drafted by winners of the six previous years, but proposed greater opportunities in government for women. He would follow it up with an order to agencies to improve the status of their G-girls.

Unfortunately, the government sometimes fails to make full use of the proven talents of its women employees. Take the case of Dr Frances Oldham Kelsey, who is Uncle Sam's most honored woman employee. It was Mrs Kelsey who blocked the sale in this country of the sleep-inducing drug thalidomide that produced malformed babies.

Several years ago the Food and Drug Administration couldn't do enough for Mrs Kelsey, its most distinguished employee. It promoted her to an administrative post, which didn't turn out to be the added recognition intended for her. About a year ago the agency began to reorganize, and she was shuffled out of that post.

Much worse, she was given what her friends say was a humiliating 'bare-desk' treatment; she was generally ignored and was given little to do of consequence.

But now she's busy and happy again. She's back at her old stand investigating drugs, and their possible harmful effects on humans ... 'My desk was pretty bare for a while, and my morale was quite low', she told friends at the awards dinner. 'But I guess those things happen to lots of people during the reorganization of their agencies'. She isn't convinced that they are necessary however.

Frankie shares a personal reminiscence in a memo to John Swann, FDA historian. In this memo, dated 26 September 1995, Frankie recalls correcting examinations with one hand and with the other rocking her daughter Christine's cradle. Frankie explains that at that time, Dr Geiling was the National Board Examiner for Pharmacology. His staff would assist him by suggesting suitable essay questions, and they earned a little much-needed extra money by grading the examinations.

A notification of a dinner at the Cosmos Club, dated 8 February 1963, says:

> We are honored to have as our speaker Frances Oldham Kelsey, MD, Chief, Investigational Drug Branch, Division of New Drugs, Bureau of Medicine, US Food and Drug Administration. Her subject is 'The investigation of new drugs'.

To quote *The Saturday Review* (1 September) [presumably 1962]:

> As everyone who can read or hear surely knows by now, Dr Kelsey is a Canadian-born medical officer of the US Food and Drug Administration who refused to approve American marketing of thalidomide, a hypnotic that somehow makes armless, legless and other monstrous cripples of babies born to women who take the drug 'to get a good night's sleep' during early pregnancy.

Here is another glimpse of Frankie's life after her great triumph over thalidomide. This is a letter to Frankie from a Caroline Swann (no relation to Dr John Swann) on 3 August 1962. The first paragraph of the letter reads:

Dear Dr Kelsey,

It was stimulating talking with you yesterday. Thank you for listening to me and for saying that you would not make another commitment until we have had the opportunity to talk out the program I outlined on the telephone. That is an exploration into the various communications media – television, motion pictures, theater – of a drama based on your life. I would have expected you to be as modest as you were when you said you did not think there was anything of great interest about your life except for the present situation. As I told you, I believe that the best dramas do not present a long biographical stand that observes Aristotle's unity. The biography is the background to the climactic story which flares out in the dramatic situation such as we have at present.

The letter continues with information about Caroline Swann's experience relevant to her proposal to produce a story based on Frankie's life. This letter, which clearly reflects the conversation Caroline Swann had with Frankie on the phone, provides an important nugget about how Frankie saw herself when she told Caroline that she didn't think there was anything of great interest about her life except for the present situation – i.e., her involvement with the thalidomide story. This is yet more evidence that Frankie was reluctant to see herself as a heroine.

The archive of Frankie's papers at the Library of Congress in Washington is a wonderfully eclectic mix of formality and informality. The formality consists of government memos and newspaper reports, while the informality is embodied in letters written to her by citizens of the United States and other countries thanking her for her work.

On 6 December 1962, Weber F. Trout, the news feature editor of the *United Press International*, wrote to Frankie to tell her that she had been named 'Woman of the Year' for her work in connection with the thalidomide affair. The letter went on to say:

We select a top woman and man of each year (JFK is the man of 1962) and carry extensive profiles on them on the countrywide trunk, which goes into about 2,500 radio and television stations.

The press release about Frankie receiving this award was not especially flattering to start with. It reminds us that back in 1962 women tended to be viewed by men as women first and people second.

> She is a plain woman ... tall and big-boned, with no makeup to cover the sharp, severe lines of her face. Her greying hair is cut straight and short – almost masculine. Her favorite outfit is a subdued tweed suit and flat-soled Oxford shoes.
>
> Dr Frances Oldham Kelsey looks like anything but a newsmaker – but first impressions are deceiving. She fought a stubborn, lonely battle ... and emerged the victor.

The remainder of this press release summarizes Frankie's life story and her work on the thalidomide case.

Frankie received numerous citations of honor, invitations to dinners, and certificates attesting to her excellence from all sorts of organizations, including her own neighbors' organization, the Kenwood Citizens Association, which said as follows:

Citation of Honor to Dr Frances O. Kelsey

For your professional skill and courage in preventing the distribution of thalidomide in this country, which was an immeasurable service rendered to your country and to the world in preventing the birth of malformed infants. In this work you enjoyed the strong support and good counsel of your husband, Dr F. Ellis Kelsey.

Your friends and neighbors in Kenwood have greatly admired your outstanding capabilities, who wish to add their sincere congratulations to the many honors you have received. We are deeply proud that one of our neighbors has so worthily earned the gratitude of our entire country.

Presented by the Kenwood Citizens Association at its dinner meeting October 22, 1962.

A letter dated 12 July 1973, to Dr Julius M. Toon, professor and chairman of the Department of Pharmacology at the Jefferson Medical College of Thomas Jefferson University in Philadelphia, gives a glimpse into Frankie's family life after her immortal achievements in safeguarding the United States against thalidomide.

The girls and I are off next week to cruise with the Fayley's in Maine. I'm afraid they acquired a very green crew. I may be able to recount our experiences if you attend the Internal Analgesics Committee meeting at the end of the month.

Best to you and Liz.

It seems that Frankie's reference to the 'Internal Analgesics Committee meeting' is an example of her sense of humor at work: no doubt she envisaged that then she would still be suffering from the effects of seasickness.

Here is a letter written by Mrs J. Seward Johnson Jr on 4 August 1962, addressed to Frankie:

Dear Dr Kelsey,

Enclosed please find a photograph of my baby daughter who may owe her life to you.

You have not only saved many of our children, but you have also set an example to them. Your persistence and courage in adhering to what you knew was right, against tremendous pressure, is an example for all of us. Please find a check enclosed made out to you. If it is possible to use this money in any way to ensure that other tragedies of this sort can be averted where persons of your stature are not in control, I would be most grateful.

Sincerely yours,

Barbara Johnson

The amount of money Barbara sent to Frankie, which of course Frankie promptly donated to the FDA, is not known as far as we are aware. Frankie replied to Barbara's letter, although the reply does not seem to have survived. If it did, it would have ended up with Barbara rather than in the FDA archive. Barbara responded to that reply on 25 August 1962:

> Dear Dr Kelsey,
> I was very happy to receive your letter of August 15. In the meantime, I have received a very nice letter from Dr Taussig supplementing your description of the purpose [for] which my money will be used, and I am most grateful to you for forwarding my contribution so that it can be spent so perfectly in accordance with my feelings.

There is a letter in the FDA archive dated 29 January 1963, Frankie's reply to George McGovern. The text is as follows:

> The Honorable George McGovern
> United States Senate
> Washington 25 DC
>
> Dear Senator McGovern,
> Thank you very much indeed for your letter of January 11, 1963. I appreciated very much your kind comments on my recent appointment. I would indeed enjoy having lunch with you some day and [reminiscing] about South Dakota.
> Sincerely yours,
> Frances O. Kelsey, MD
> Chief, Investigational Drug Branch
> Division of New Drugs
> Bureau of Medicine

In some letters in the archive, it's not entirely clear how serious or tongue-in-cheek Frankie is being. For example, on 1 June 1967, Frankie writes a letter to a Mike Myers of Minnesota.

Dear Mike,

I must apologize for being a little late in answering your recent letter of enquiry as to my opinion on flying saucers. This, however, is a subject in which I have done no research and have no first-time information and would have very little to offer.

Sincerely yours,

Frances O. Kelsey, MD

Frankie's fame continued to grow. She became known and loved around the world for the role she had played in saving tens of thousands of American children from the scourge of thalidomide.

Frankie's sense of humor rarely deserted her. On 27 May 1998, when she was 84 years old, she sent John Swann a handwritten memo regarding a letter she had received, an example of the famous 'advanced fees scam' in which a recipient is promised an enormous amount of money if he or she will allow the funds to be transferred to their bank account. Once they agree, they are simply asked for advanced fees to cover expenses, and of course the whole point of the scam is to collect these advanced fees. There is never any actual money available to the person being scammed. In this case the supposed group executive director of a large Nigerian oil company offered Frankie a share of very substantial proceeds if she would initiate a business relationship with them in order to transfer funds into her account.

This proposal found no reception with Frankie at all; her handwritten memo to John Swann reads: *For your amusement. An offer I did not act on!*

The letter was addressed to Frankie at the Office of Compliance at the FDA. Obviously her fame had reached as far as Nigeria, and someone there thought that the woman who had spent a crucial fourteen months of her life defending the United States from thalidomide might be gullible enough to fall victim to the scam. Needless to say, that didn't wash with our heroine.

Frankie received well-deserved plaudits, congratulations, and awards from all around the world. In her archive at the Library of Congress, there are thick files full of heartwarming letters of congratulations from people who knew Frankie, and similar letters from many more who didn't. Just one example of a letter from a stranger comes from a Miss L. Lawson, who says:

Dear Dr Kelsey,
I pray God that there may be more dedicated doctors like you.

Frankie continued to work for the FDA while her magnificent work was being more and more widely recognized. She was still working at the FDA's Center for Drug Evaluation and Research in 1995 and was appointed deputy for scientific and medical affairs. In 1994, the Frances Kelsey Secondary School in Mill Bay, British Columbia, was named in her honor. Frankie retired from the FDA in 2005.

Dr John Swann recalls that Frankie enjoyed playing golf in her retirement and had a very sharp mind, but she gradually began to have problems driving and so had to stop using her car. John used to visit her and have coffee and sherry with her. She only retired in 2005, aged 87, and went home in 2014 to live in Ontario with her daughter Christine. As John says: 'Frances didn't dwell on what she'd done. Other people made more of it than she did'.

In 2010, the FDA presented Frankie with the first Drug Safety Excellence Award and named the annual award after her, announcing that it would be given to one FDA staff member annually.

America's largest Catholic newspaper, *Catholic New York,* contained an article on 23 September 2010, by Claudia McDonnell about Frankie. It read:

One of my heroes was honored last week. I hadn't seen her name in a long time until I happened to pick up a newspaper article that told the story.

I suspect that many people have never heard of her, but I have admired Dr Frances Oldham Kelsey since I was a girl.

It's been almost fifty years since she made front-page news, but she deserves to be known and remembered, because she prevented what would almost certainly have been a wave of birth defects affecting thousands of children and families. She saved them from the drug thalidomide, which caused so much harm in Europe. She had to buck powerful people and withstand a lot criticism to do it, but she held her ground. Later she was vindicated and honored, and now, at age ninety-six, she has been honored again.

The article continues:

Dr Kelsey's work led to the passage of a law that gave the FDA stronger control over drug testing and regulation. Dr Kelsey and her colleagues established new rules for drug testing that are now used worldwide.

Dr Kelsey received the President's Award for Distinguished Federal Civilian Service from President John F. Kennedy in 1962. She was honored by the University of Chicago, and in 2000 she was inducted into the National Women's Hall of Fame in Seneca Falls. On September 15 she became the first recipient of a new award to be given annually by the FDA to one of its staff members: the Doctor Frances O. Kelsey Award for Excellence and Courage in Protecting Public Health.

Claudia McDonnell concludes the article by saying:

I admire Dr Kelsey for her discipline as a scientist and her commitment to her profession. Even more, I admire the moral courage of this woman who could not be bullied, who was faithful to her responsibility, who suffered harassment and would not compromise. She set a shining example.

Frankie had her 100th birthday on 24 July 2014. The following day a party was held for her at the Cosmos Club. The bill for the party was

$2,249.61. It's not clear whether Frankie paid this bill herself, but we think she probably did.

In one of the most wonderful plaudits accorded to Frankie on her birthday, then governor-general of Canada, David Johnston, wrote to her in the following terms:

> Dear Dr Kelsey,
>
> Birthdays are an occasion to reflect upon life's many joys, all of which form who we are today. It is a chance to celebrate the accomplishments we have made through hard work and determination, the wisdom we have gained through experience and, most importantly, the elite people we have met along the way of this incredible journey.
>
> Over the years, you have experienced the world's many cycles and revolutions of change; your own personal history is forever woven into the tapestry of Canadian heritage.
>
> It is therefore my pleasure to join your family and friends in wishing you a very happy one hundredth birthday, as well as many more years of happiness.
>
> Yours sincerely,
>
> David Johnston
>
> Governor-General of Canada

Frankie received many other tributes on her hundredth birthday, including an unforgettable one from the legendary Sir Harold ('Harry') Evans, who was editor of *The Sunday Times* from 1967 to 1981. He was the instigator, figurehead, and leader of the highly successful *Sunday Times* campaign to win proper compensation for thalidomide sufferers in the United Kingdom. As Sir Harry wrote to Frankie:

> Dear Dr Kelsey
>
> You are only one hundred but you saved many, many hundreds of thousands of your fellow human beings from cruel lives and early death.

The application in 1960 for FDA approval of Kevadon (alias thalidomide) was your first case at the agency. Ten million pills had already been produced by a major pharmaceutical company for distribution throughout the United States. They assumed that approval would come, as it had elsewhere around the world. You were not to know the catastrophic teratogenic effect of thalidomide, no one did then. Your heroism was twofold: one, in your insistence on the primacy of scientific evidence; two, in your courage in the face of incessant pressure from powerful interests.

This is what prevented the massacre of the innocent in the United States. At *The Sunday Times* in London, when we began investigating the origins of thalidomide, the greatest drug tragedy ever known, moved as we were by the injustice of families left to cope, we were inspired through many long years of prosecution and suppression by your shining example.

It would have been a signal achievement just to prevent thalidomide creating the havoc in the Unites States that it did around the world. You did that, but by your integrity and your courage you also testified to the endurable virtue of truth.

This deeply moving testimony from Sir Harry aptly summarizes many of Frankie's achievements, but it's important we point out, with great deference to Sir Harry, that it is not accurate that she had no inkling of thalidomide's teratogenic effect before it was revealed. As we've seen, she did suspect this.

Frankie's good friend J. Richard Crout sent her a birthday card and a letter for her centenary birthday. His letter reads as follows:

Dear Frances,

I would love to be at your luncheon today but am in Michigan on vacation. I will be thinking of you and wishing I could give you a personal hug. I enjoyed so much working with you at FDA. Beyond your thalidomide decision that is so honored, and properly so, you brought continuing lifelong leadership, expertise and common sense to our entire new drug review process, our toxicology programs in teratology, and our entire clinical investigations program. And beyond that, you gave to everyone in the Agency your example of grace under pressure and allegiance to the evidence and the truth.

So to some you may be the Queen (a good title, no doubt), but to me you will always be Madame Integrity. I am particularly grateful for your friendship, support, and [encouragment] during some trying times at [the] FDA. I look back on those days with great respect and affection. Now you have given me another gift: the chance to honor your one hundredth birthday. Once again you are showing us the best it can be. May the day be beautiful for you, surrounded by friends and family. May your future be bright and filled with happiness.

With admiration and love,

Dick Crout

J. Richard Crout adds this on the card he sent Frankie:

Wherever you go, no matter how far the journey, know that I'm thinking of you, and the light you shine. Happy Birthday. Dick. PS: I am well and only eighty-nine.

Sixteen

LAST DAYS

Shortly after turning 100, in the autumn of 2014, Frankie moved from Washington, D.C., to live with her daughter Christine in London, Ontario.

In June 2015, when Frankie was named to the Order of Canada, Mercédes Benegbi, the then head of the Thalidomide Victims Association of Canada, praised Frankie for showing strength and courage by refusing to bend to pressure from drug company officials. He said, 'To us, she was always our heroine, even if what she did was in another country'.

Frankie passed away peacefully in London, Ontario, on 7 August 2015, at the age of 101. Few human lives have been lived as well, or as long, as hers. Less than twenty-four hours earlier, Ontario's lieutenant-governor, Elizabeth Dowdeswell, had visited Frankie at home to present her with the insignia of Member of the Order of Canada for her important role in defending the babies, children, and parents of the United States against thalidomide.

Frankie's life was a life of quiet, arduous, meticulous work. She never saw herself as a heroine, but she was. In this sense she was a reluctant heroine, and perhaps, ultimately, reluctant heroes and heroines are the most heroic of all. After Frankie's achievement became known, she won hearts all over the world. Those hearts are a great testament to her life's work.

Without her work, her adherence to her professional principles, her love of science and the objectivity that science brings, and her passion for carrying out her public duties as a servant of the United States government and of its people, there is no doubt that tens of thousands of households throughout the US would have been afflicted with unborn children who died in the womb or were born with all kinds of health problems and deformities.

The story of thalidomide really does show human beings at their worst and at their best. Yes, it is a story of selfishness, greed, short-sightedness, ignorance, wickedness, and lack of imagination on the part of the men who developed and were so eager to market their 'wonder drug' around the world. But while human beings can be all those things, they can also be so much more: selfless, caring, visionary, wise, compassionate and good, loving, imaginative, and everything else that is wonderful about people. Above all, Frankie's story is the story of her deep and abiding love for the people she was professionally committed to protect, and how she protected them with all her energy, might and courage.

EPILOGUE

Dr Kelsey is no longer with us, but her life and achievement continue to resonate in our world.

The powerful play *[Miss]* by US playwright W.L. Newkirk was first produced in 2016 and won the Charles M. Getchell Award as the Best New Play of 2017. The name of the play includes the brackets Dr Stehle suggested that Frankie put on her application letter. *[Miss]* tells the story of the Kelsey–Merrell confrontation. The play has been very well received and had a highly successful run at the Orlando Shakespeare Center in 2017. The first act of the play was published in the Autumn 2017 issue of *Southern Theater* magazine, while the second is available for reading online at www.setc.org/miss. The following extract is reproduced by kind permission of the playwright.

(Phone rings. Lights up on KELSEY on the phone. MURRAY answers.)
Hello.
KELSEY: Dr Murray.
MURRAY: Dr Kelsey. Hello.

KELSEY: They told me you'd been calling.

MURRAY: For days.

KELSEY: I'm sorry. It's taking me a while to learn the ropes.

MURRAY: I thought you'd fallen off the face of the earth.

KELSEY: Nope. Still here, unfortunately.

MURRAY: Well, you've got us all in suspense. What's the verdict? *(Long pause.)* Dr Kelsey? You still there?

KELSEY: You should have your application back –

MURRAY: Back?

KELSEY: In a few days.

MURRAY: So, you approved it?

KELSEY: No.

MURRAY: You rejected it?

KELSEY: No.

MURRAY: What're you doing then?

KELSEY: Returning it.

MURRAY: Returning it?! Why?!

KELSEY: It's. *(Beat. KELSEY thinks.)* Incomplete.

MURRAY: It's. Incomplete? How?

KELSEY: Well, you cite a lot of German studies.

MURRAY: It's a German drug.

KELSEY: But, your German translations are – wrong.

MURRAY: You cannot be serious.

KELSEY: I am. Get a better translator.

MURRAY: *(Beat. Getting his bearings.)* Anything else?

KELSEY: You include thirty reports from American doctors.

MURRAY: Our investigational study.

KELSEY: These aren't even *remotely* an investigational study. They're *testimonials.*

MURRAY: They're a study.

KELSEY: To be honest, most of them are barely believable.

MURRAY: You don't like them?

KELSEY: It's not a matter of *liking* them. You need real studies.

MURRAY: Anything else?

KELSEY: Your rats.

MURRAY: Let me guess: You want them to die.

KELSEY: Rats have trouble absorbing certain drugs.

MURRAY: So, now you're an expert on rats?

KELSEY: Actually, I am.

MURRAY: Unbelievable!

KELSEY: And if you want to give Kevadon to pregnant women –

MURRAY: You know we do –

KELSEY: Provide us with research that shows Kevadon's safe in pregnancy.

MURRAY: You done?

KELSEY: No, there's a few more.

MURRAY: I'm sure.

KELSEY: I can put them in the cover letter, if you'd like.

MURRAY: That'd be great.

KELSEY: Fine. Let us know if you want to resubmit.

MURRAY: Oh, we will.

KELSEY: Bye.

(*KELSEY hangs up and gives a big sigh of relief. MURRAY looks at the phone. Lights out over KELSEY. MURRAY gets up. Starts to pace. Furious.*)

POGGE: You OK?

MURRAY: Apparently, we can't translate German.

POGGE: *What?!*

MURRAY: (*Explodes*) *DAMMIT! THERE GOES CHRISTMAS!*

POGGE: No way she turned us down.

MURRAY: She didn't.

POGGE: So, what's the problem?

MURRAY: She's *returning* our application.

POGGE: Can she even *do* that, legally?

MURRAY: She thinks she can.

POGGE: Doesn't she know how the game is played?

MURRAY: Apparently not.

POGGE: Bitch!

(Pause. They think.)

POGGE: We gotta crush her.

MURRAY: I'll start making some calls.

POGGE: Who?

MURRAY: Public Relations to start.

POGGE: Those PR guys'll make her wish she never heard of Kevadon.

MURRAY: And. We apply again.

POGGE: What d'ya need from me?

MURRAY: Research.

POGGE: She's already got the German stuff.

MURRAY: *American.* American research. American docs. American journals.

POGGE: That's gonna take time.

MURRAY: And a study on pregnancy.

POGGE: Pregnancy?

MURRAY: That shows Kevadon is safe.

POGGE: I might have someone for that.

MURRAY: Who?

POGGE: Ray Nulsen.

MURRAY: Never heard of him.

POGGE: He was Don Merrell's fraternity brother.

MURRAY: Is he sharp?

POGGE: Let's just say: He'll be very cooperative and geographically convenient.

MURRAY: Good.

Why exactly did thalidomide cause so much damage to babies' bodies in the first place?

While the precise mechanism by which thalidomide causes deformities and other damage to the bodies of unborn children is still not completely understood, today the general consensus is that it influences human

DNA in a way that leads to an anti-angiogenic effect. This means that thalidomide inhibits the formation of small blood vessels in unborn fetuses. There have been more than two thousand research papers published about the teratogenic action of thalidomide and about fifteen possible and plausible mechanisms have been suggested. However, the most likely one seems to be that it slows and prevents the formation of small blood vessels in the very young fetus, which in practice means up to about forty-six days after conception. One paper has stated:

Loss of newly-formed blood vessels is the primary cause of thalidomide teratogenesis, and developing limbs are particularly susceptible because of their relatively immature, highly angiogenic vessel network.

Most likely thalidomide has other effects as well. In particular, it is known to bind to an inactive protein called cereblon, which is important in limb formation development in the fetus and also causes the proliferation of myeloma cells.

The old saying 'It's an ill wind that blows nobody any good' implies that even very bad events can have some positive consequences. In the case of thalidomide, the very toxicity of the drug to the unborn fetus has turned out to have positive benefits for some illnesses that can be improved – for instance, if blood flow at the bodily extremities is restricted in some way.

In particular, thalidomide has been found to be helpful in treating some forms of leprosy. In 1964, Israeli physician Jacob Sheskis administered it to a patient who was critically ill with a condition called erythema nodosum leprosum (ENL), a painful skin condition and one of the complications of leprosy. This was attempted despite the ban on thalidomide's use, but results were favorable. The patient slept for hours and was soon able to get out of bed without aid upon waking up. A clinical trial studying the use of thalidomide in leprosy soon followed and it has been used by Brazilian doctors as the drug of choice for the treatment of severe ENL since 1965.

Unfortunately, despite rigid prohibitions on giving the treatment to pregnant women, by 1996 at least thirty-three cases of embryos damaged by thalidomide had been recorded in people born in Brazil after 1965. Since 1994, production, dispensing and prescription has been strictly controlled, requiring women who are taking it to use two forms of birth control and submit to regular pregnancy tests. Despite this, cases of thalidomide embryopathy continue, with at least one hundred cases identified in Brazil between 2005 and 2010. During these five years, 5.8 million thalidomide pills were distributed throughout Brazil, largely to poor Brazilians in areas with poor access to healthcare.

Thalidomide was finally approved by the FDA in 1998. Frankie was brought in from retirement in order to supervise the approval process. In the United States, thalidomide is only authorized for use in the treatment of ENL, and because of its potential for causing birth defects, the drug may be distributed only under tightly controlled conditions. The FDA required that the Celgene Corporation, which planned to market the drug under the brand name Thalomid, establish a system for thalidomide education and prescribing safety. The conditions required under the program include limiting prescription and dispensing rights to authorized prescribers in pharmacies only, keeping a database of all patients with prescriptions for thalidomide, providing extensive patient education about the risks associated with the drug, and providing periodic pregnancy tests for women who take the drug. In 2010, the World Health Organization (WHO) stated that it did not recommend thalidomide due to the difficulty of adequately controlling its use.

Thalidomide has also been found to be beneficial in treating patients with multiple myeloma for whom standard treatments have failed. Again, the effectiveness of the drug against multiple myeloma appears to be due to its ability to inhibit the formation of blood vessels, something which is desirable in controlling this disease. Multiple myeloma, also known as plasma cell myeloma, is a cancer of the plasma cells, the type of white blood cell normally responsible for producing antibodies. Often initially no symptoms of multiple myeloma are noticed. When advanced, bone pain, bleeding, frequent infections, and anemia may occur. Multiple myeloma usually has a five-year survival rate of 49 per cent. Without treatment, typical survival is seven months, but with treatment, survival is usually four to five years.

Thalidomide is now used worldwide as a treatment for multiple myeloma, but as always great caution is taken to ensure that women who are taking the drug do not get pregnant. The expiration of the anti-angiogenic and immunomodulatory properties of thalidomide had led to the study and creation of a thalidomide analogue. In pharmacology, a drug analogue is a compound having a structure similar to that of the drug, but differing from it in respect of at least one component. The organization Celgene has sponsored numerous clinical trials with analogues to thalidomide such as lenalidomide, which is significantly more powerful, has fewer side effects, and offers greater myelosuppression. The analogues still have teratogenic effects, however.

The irony is that thalidomide is a potent treatment for some very unpleasant conditions, including cancers. It was initially launched as a powerful sedative without any side effects; in fact its side effects are disastrous, but it does have some important curative properties. But no one, least of all Merrell, knew that back in September 1960, when the thalidomide NDA was launched.

Another irony is that, essentially, Frankie saved Merrell. If thalidomide had been authorized for distribution throughout the United States, Merrell certainly would have been bankrupted – many times over – by the vast number of lawsuits that would have resulted. As a Merrell lawyer subsequently and accurately remarked, 'If it hadn't been for her, we'd be out of business'.

The first British thalidomide babies were born in January 1959, but it would be nearly three years before Grünenthal, the Germany drug company that developed the drug, acknowledged the connection. By then, ten thousand babies had been born worldwide.

In 1968 UK manufacturer Distillers Biochemicals Limited (now part of the organization Diageo) reached a compensation settlement for babies born with thalidomide problems following a legal battle by the families they had affected. In 1972 *The Sunday Times* published a front page lead story with the headline 'Our Thalidomide Children, a Cause for National Shame', part of a long-running campaign for further compensation for thalidomide-affected children, as the initial settlement from Distillers was not particularly generous. Eventually a total of £28 million was paid out by Diageo during the 1970s.

Lynette Rowe, a Melbourne woman who was born without limbs, led an Australian class action lawsuit against the drug's manufacturer, Grünenthal, that fought to have the case heard in Germany. The Supreme Court of Victoria dismissed Grünenthal's application in 2012, and the case was heard in Australia.

On 17 July 2012, Rowe was awarded an out-of-court settlement, believed to be in the millions of dollars and paving the way for class action victims to receive further compensation. In February 2014, the Supreme Court of Victoria endorsed the settlement of AU$80 million to 107 victims of the drug in Australia and New Zealand.

Many people affected by thalidomide have achieved great career success. There are too many to list here, but here are a few:

Lorraine Mercer MBE of the United Kingdom. Born with phocomelia of both arms and legs, she is the only thalidomide survivor to carry the Olympic Torch. Lorraine's motto is 'No Limbs, No Limits!'

Nico von Glasow, born with disabilities due to thalidomide, is an eminent German movie director and producer.

Thomas Quasthoff is an internationally acclaimed bass-baritone. A thalidomide survivor, he describes himself as '1.34 meters tall, short arms, seven fingers – four right, three left – large, relatively well-formed head, brown eyes, distinctive lips; profession: singer'.

Kev Donnellon says:

Those of us who have been affected by thalidomide call ourselves 'thalidomiders'. We're proud to call ourselves that. We see ourselves, rightly enough, as belonging to a select and exceptional community. Most of us thalidomiders have been on TV and radio, and we've appeared in newspapers on countless occasions. Being a unique group of people, our lives have been scrutinized in the media.

This isn't to say that we thalidomiders seek public attention or fame. Ideally many of us would, I think, like to keep ourselves to ourselves, but that's not how our lives turned out ... .

People often tell us they find us inspiring. Well, I suppose if you do have proper arms and proper legs, and understandably can't readily imagine not having them, you might find someone who doesn't have arms and legs but somehow manages to cope with life, inspiring in some way. I imagine, too, that it can be helpful to think of me when, for example, you're lying nice and snug in bed on a cold winter morning with a difficult day at work ahead of you and you feel a bit daunted by the idea of having to get up. At that moment you could perhaps give yourself some real impetus to get up and hop into the shower by thinking to yourself, for example, *Come on, get up! Kev doesn't even have any legs or arms, and he manages to get up and out of the house on a cold winter morning, and you're lucky enough to have arms and legs, so just get up and start using them!*

If you do find my story inspirational in that respect or in any other way, I'm glad. The truth is, though, that I've never really set out to inspire anybody – I've just got on with my life.

And then there is the charismatic Mandy Masters from Britain.

My name is Mandy Masters, [and] I'm a fifty-six-year-old woman and a strong survivor of thalidomide. I was born without arms and use my feet just like you use your hands. I've been happily married for thirty-seven years with a wonderful hubby, two daughters, and eight grandsons. Having my family is like building my cake, and the cherry on the top was my grandchildren. I'm a very well-known columnist in a well-known monthly magazine. I've been a makeup artist and worked on a switchboard in my earlier days. I've never let my disability stop me doing anything. My parents loved me from day one and brought me up to live a normal and happy life, and that's what I do. I'm now known to many as their walking Earth Angel. My dream now would be to have my own chat show or be on a British TV program called *Loose Women*. The doctors gave my parents a bleak future for me and basically said I would be a cabbage. Well, I guess they got that wrong!

THE END

Appendix One

SAFETY OF DRUGS DURING PREGNANCY

BY FRANCES O. KELSEY, PHD, MD

(Presented to the International Childbirth Education Association Eastern Regional Conference of 1967, sponsored by Materna, Friday, 21 April 1967, International Inn, Washington, D.C.)

It is a well-recognized fact that no drug is completely without hazard and that before one is administered to human subjects, the benefits expected from the drug must be carefully weighed against the possible risks entailed by its administration.

When drugs are administered during pregnancy, two evaluations must be reached: that involving the safety to the mother; and that involving the safety to the unborn child.

In reviewing current knowledge in this area, consideration will be given not only to the effects on the unborn child of drugs given to the mother, but also to the effects of drugs on the newborn, particularly the premature newborn; whether these drugs are given to the offspring itself or whether they reach the offspring through the mother, as for example, drugs given to the mother shortly before delivery, or drugs that may reach a nursing offspring following excretion in the mother's milk.

Until comparatively recently it was felt that the placenta served as a protective barrier preventing exposure of the embryo to drugs and other compounds consumed by the mother during pregnancy. We now know that the so-called placental barrier permits virtually all such substances to pass from the mother's bloodstream to that of the developing child. It is true that a few are sufficiently large, or have other properties that interfere with their passage across the placental barrier. Nevertheless, even these substances may enter the fetal circulation under certain circumstances, as for example, if they are present in high concentrations or if the placenta is damaged by disease or other circumstances.

We now know that the developing child does not deal with a drug in the same way that the adult does. It does not have as efficient mechanisms for elimination of toxic substances from the body and it lacks many of the intricate enzymatic processes by which the cells of the adult detoxify ingested substances. We also know that substances need not cross the placental barrier to have an effect on the fetus, but may exert an indirect effect by interfering with the metabolic processes of the mother.

There is also reason to believe that pregnancy may alter the ability of the mother to detoxify drugs, an effect which could mean additional hazard to both mother and child. A possible example of this is the apparent increased risk of liver and kidney toxicity when tetracycline is given in late pregnancy.

Once a drug has passed through the placental barrier, its effect on the developing child may depend on a number of factors, the most striking being the time at which a drug is given. Drugs given very early in pregnancy may result in death of the embryo and subsequent abortion which may or may not be recognized. Drugs given during the period of the rapid development of the organ-systems of the embryo, if the drug is not sufficiently toxic to cause death, may give rise to distortions of growth which result in birth deformities. In either case, the adverse effect on the fetus may be elicited by doses of the drug that are quite harmless to the mother. Drugs given to the mother later in pregnancy may produce effects on the fetus that resemble their known toxic effects in the adult, or in some cases, the effects may be more or less unique to the offspring.

With regard to examples of drugs known to be harmful if given during pregnancies, consideration will first be given to those whose administration has been associated with teratogenic activity.

While the thalidomide episode has been largely credited with drawing attention to the hazards of drugs during pregnancy, the association between birth defects and drugs, infections, or other environmental factors had been recognized for some years. Thus, in 1929, Murphy reported microcephaly and mental retardation in a high per cent of offspring of mothers receiving pelvic irradiation during pregnancy. Similar malformations were reported in offspring of mothers who were exposed to the atomic bomb explosion in Hiroshima in 1945, In 1941, a second environmental factor was recognized as the cause of congenital malformation when Gregg, in Australia, reported that German measles in the first trimester of pregnancy was frequently associated with congenital malformations in the offspring. Gregg's studies have been repeatedly confirmed and recent studies would indicate that perhaps 15 per cent of children whose mothers were exposed to measles during the first sixteen weeks of pregnancy have severe congenital anomalies including eye damage, hearing loss, and heart defects, while another 16 per cent may have minor congenital anomalies.

In 1952, Thiersch reported that the drug aminopterin used in the treatment of leukemia frequently resulted in deaths or deformities in the offspring of women receiving the drug early in pregnancy.

We now know that most, if not all, drugs that are presently useful in the treatment of cancer do carry the hazard of causing deformities in the offspring if used during pregnancy. However, a number of women have been treated throughout pregnancy with these drugs and have given birth to apparently perfectly normal children. In the treatment of cancer during pregnancy, the physician must weigh the risk to the infant against possible benefits to the mother. However, some of these drugs are used in less serious conditions, such as psoriasis or rheumatoid arthritis, and in patients with these conditions it would seem unjustifiable to use the drug if the pregnancy were established or suspected.

Another group of drugs associated with congenital malformations include certain steroid natural and synthetic hormone preparations. Progestational agents in high doses have long been advocated in threatened abortion and an appreciable number of mothers receiving these preparations have given birth to female offspring with masculanization of the external genitalia. This effect has also been reported in the offspring of a patient who self-administered a geriatric vitamin-hormone preparation obtained from a neighbor during pregnancy. None of the affected girls have, as of this year, yet reached the childbearing age, so that the full significance of the defect cannot be evaluated. While seldom requiring surgery, it does present a severe emotional problem. In addition, the condition must be distinguished from the more serious forms of masculanization due to disorders of the adrenal or pituitary glands which require prompt and vigorous attention.

A number of other compounds have been implicated as causing congenital defects. It is often very difficult, however, to establish a cause-and-effect relationship. While estimates vary, the figure commonly cited is that approximately 2 per cent of all living children have defects recognizable at birth, and the figure is doubled during the first year of life, since many deformities are not readily recognizable in the newborn. Probably less than 20 per cent of the birth deformities can be accounted for by genetic factors, and known environmental hazards, including x-irradiation, certain infections, and certain drugs. To establish a relationship between the intake of a given drug and a recorded birth defect, is a formidable process, because of the relatively high per cent of these defects which occur for as yet unknown causes. In order to establish that a drug caused, for example, a 5-per cent instance of malformation when given during pregnancy, would require the study of some 1,500 pregnancies in which half, or 750, mothers received the drug and the other half did not. It is readily apparent that this type of data is not available for the vast majority of drugs that may be administered to women during pregnancy.

A few examples may now be cited of drugs recognized as being hazardous to the infant when given to the mother during the later stages of pregnancy. It is now well established that offspring born to narcotic addicts may show evidence of morphine addiction at birth, including pin-point pupils and depressed respiration. More importantly, they may suffer severe and fatal withdrawal symptoms unless the condition is promptly recognized and appropriately treated. This adverse effect has also been reported as a result of the prescribing during pregnancy of a morphine-like compound for the treatment of ulcerative colitis. Again, goiter may be present in the newborn child whose mother has been given thyroid-suppressing compounds such as thiouracil preparations; or iodide preparations, such as may be given for asthma. These goiters may be sufficiently large as to interfere with delivery of the child or may cause breathing difficulties or actual suffocation. They rapidly subside after the birth of the baby results in removal from exposure to the drug. However, it is important that these goiters be recognized as drug-induced, since they will usually require no treatment other than supportive measures. Anticoagulant drugs such as the dicumarol and phenindione preparations may cause serious or even fatal bleeding in the developing child if given to the mother.

The preceding examples illustrate toxic effects readily recognizable as being drug induced since they resemble the adverse effects that may occur in adults. Additionally, because the developing embryo or the newborn cannot always handle drugs as does the adult, certain types of toxic reactions may be seen in the young that are seldom, if ever, seen in the adult. A striking example of this is the dray syndrome, characterized by circulatory collapse and often death in premature babies given chloramphenicol in doses comparable to those used in the adult. It is now known that the liver of the baby lacks the processes that the adult has for rendering the antibiotic less toxic. By giving the newborn babies dosages much smaller in comparison to the adult, this toxicity can be avoided.

Again, a number of compounds may cause jaundice in the newborn if given to the mother before birth, or to the child shortly after birth, particularly if the child is premature. Compounds particularly liable to cause this jaundice include the long-acting sulfanilamide preparations, certain vitamin K preparations, the antibiotic novobiocin and various salicylate preparations. There are a number of mechanisms that may cause this jaundice, but the net results are the same. The concern is that bile pigment, bilirubin, the cause of the jaundice, may diffuse into the brain and be deposited there giving rise to the so-called 'kernicterus' which may be associated with mental retardation or even death of the child.

As a final example, heart lesions and other defects such as mental retardation may result from high blood calcium levels associated with excess vitamin D intake, either by the mother during late pregnancy or by the newborn infant.

Finally, consideration may be given to possibility of adverse effects to the infant from drugs excreted in the mother's milk. It is known that virtually all drugs will pass into the milk, the same principles applying to passage of drugs into the milk as across the placental barrier. However, little attention has been paid to the possible hazards to the nursing infant of drugs taken by the mother, and few studies have been prepared relative to the amount of any given drug that might reach the nursing child.

Strong purgatives; atrophine; and ergot preparations have long been contraindicated for nursing mothers. The oral contraceptive agents are excreted in human milk, but their effect on the nursing child is as yet undetermined. However, they may suppress lactation, and therefore are contraindicated in the nursing mother. Radioactive iodine is known to be excreted in appreciable amounts in milk and this drug, and indeed other radioisotopes, might well be avoided during lactation as well as during pregnancy.

Recently jaundice has been described in nursing infants which has been shown to be due to a breakdown product of one of the mother's steroid hormones. This is apparently a benign form of jaundice that clears up even if nursing is continued.

A severe skin disease was reported some years ago in the nursing offspring of mothers who had eaten wheat seed treated with the fungicide hexochlorobenzene. Methemoglobinemia, often associated in infants with the ingestion of well water containing high concentrations of nitrates or with absorption of dye stuffs used to mark diapers, and occasionally with the misuse of certain laundry products, was reported in a nursing infant whose mother was being treated with the anticonvulsants diphenylhydantoin and phenobarbitol.

It is well to remember that cow's milk and drinking water may also be contaminated with drugs and other environmental chemicals such as pesticides. It is the responsibility of the Food and Drug Administration to see that the presence of such substances in milk does not exceed certain levels.

Finally, it should be recognized that drugs given during pregnancy or early life may not manifest their toxicity until some later date. An obvious example of this is the staining of an infant's teeth which may result if the mother is given tetracycline during the time of tooth development. The discoloration is not observable until the teeth erupt. Again, animal experiments suggest that certain drugs given to the mother during pregnancy may affect the subsequent behavior or wellbeing of the offspring. Little or no information exists as to whether this effect may also occur in man.

Brief mention should be made of the preclinical tests that Food and Drug requires before a new drug can be administered to women capable of becoming pregnant, or to a newborn child. In the first instance, it is necessary that reproduction studies be done in at least two species of animals. For drugs administered to the newborn, the toxicity of the drug in newborn rats must be compared with that in adult animals.

While such tests may yield important information, nevertheless, it is unfortunately true that there is a wide species variation in all reactions to drugs, including adverse effects in pregnancy, and the neonatal period. While most of these studies are done in the common laboratory animals, such as the rat and rabbit, increasing attention is being paid to the possibilities that monkey and other non-human primates may yield results that would be more applicable to man. Much active research and development is being undertaken in this field and preliminary studies ... indicate that, for example, the monkey reacts to such substances as thalidomide, progestational agents, and the measles virus in a similar fashion to man.

In conclusion, consideration might be given to what steps are being taken or ... can be taken to minimize the hazard to the offspring of drugs taken by the mother during pregnancy, at the time of delivery, and during lactation. Certainly, no drug should be given during pregnancy, or indeed, at any other time unless there are specific indications for it. indeed, the most severe effects of drugs, e.g., death of the embryo or teratogenesis, may be manifested early in pregnancy at a time when the mother may not realize she is pregnant.

A problem of unknown magnitude is provided by self-administered over-the-counter preparations. Often these preparations contain a wide variety of compounds, many of which have not been tested, even in animals, for their safety in pregnancy. Often the patient does not consider them to be drugs and fails to inform her obstetrician that she has taken such a preparation. Additionally, patients may receive prescription drugs from well-meaning friends or neighbors. Again, the intake of such substances is frequently overlooked or forgotten by the time the delivery of a malformed infant occurs.

However, if the drug is prescribed or taken during pregnancy, careful records should be kept of the nature of the drug, the amount, and the date or dates or administration.

There are obviously many times during pregnancy when the withholding of a drug would have much more serious consequences than the possible risk of adverse effects to either the mother or the child, and it would, indeed, be unfortunate if fear of adverse reactions to the offspring led to the withholding of a drug that might be essential to the mother's well-being.

Appendix Two

DR FRANCES OLDHAM KELSEY'S CURRICULUM VITAE

(This is as of Frankie's retirement from the FDA in 2005.)

Frances Kathleen Oldham Kelsey, PhD, MD

Residence: 5811 Brookside Drive, Chevy Chase, Maryland 20815

Present Position: Director

Division of Scientific Investigations

Office of Compliance

Center for Drugs and Biologics

Date of Birth: 24 July 1914

Place of Birth: Cobble Hill, Vancouver Island, British Columbia, Canada

Education:			
McGill, Montreal	1934	BS
McGill, Montreal	1935	MS
University of Chicago	1938	PhD
University of Chicago	1950	MD

Memberships in Professional and Scientific Societies:

> American Society of Pharmacology and Experimental
> Therapeutics, Inc.
> American Medical Women's Association
> Congenital Anomalies Research Association of Japan
> Society for Experimental Biology and Medicine
> Sigma Xi
> New York Academy of Science
> Royal Society of Medicine
> The Teratology Society
> The European Teratology Society
> American Medical Writers Association

Awards:

> John J. Abel Fellowship
> Lederle Medical Faculty Award
> The President's Award for Distinguished Federal Civilian
> Service 1962
> Public Service Award – Association of Federal Investigators
> October 1976
> DHHS Distinguished Service Award (Scientific) 1984

Experience:

> September 1938 to September 1950, University of Chicago –
> Instructor, Then Assistant Professor
> September 1950 to September 1952, American Medical
> Association, Chicago, Illinois – Editorial Associate
> February 1953 to February 1954, Sacred Heart Hospital, Yankton,
> South Dakota – Intern
> September 1954 to September 1957, University of South
> Dakota – Associate Professor of Pharmacology
> September 1957 to 1960, Vermillion, South Dakota – General
> Practitioner

August 1960 to August 1963, FDA, Bureau of Medicine, Medical
    Officer, Washington, D.C.

August 1963 to August 1966, FDA, Bureau of Medicine, Division of
    New Drugs, Chief, Investigational Drug Branch

August 1966 to February 1967, FDA, Bureau of Medicine, Office
    of New Drugs, Director, Division of Oncology and
    Radiopharmaceutical Drug Products

February 1967 to January 1968, Assistant to the Director for Scientific
    Investigations, Bureau of Medicine, FDA

January 1968 to February 1971, Director, Division of Scientific
    Investigations, Office of Medical Support, Bureau of Medicine, FDA

February 1971 to April 1977, Director, Scientific Investigations Staff,
    Office of Scientific Evaluation, Bureau of Drugs, FDA

April 1977 to June 1982, Director, Division of Scientific Investigations,
    Office of New Drug Evaluation, Bureau of Drugs, FDA

June 1982 to Present, Director, Division of Scientific Investigations,
    Office of Compliance, Center for Drugs and Biologics

Appendix Three

PUBLICATIONS BY DR FRANCES OLDHAM KELSEY

---

1. 'The Action of the Preparations from the Posterior Lobe of the Pituitary Gland upon the Imbibition of Water by Frogs'. Frances K. Oldham, *Am. J. Physiol.* 115, 275–280 (1936).

2. 'Choline as a Factor in the Elaboration of Adrenaline'. R.L. Stehie, K.I. Melville and Frances K. Oldham, *J. Pharm. and Exper. Therap.* 56, 473–481 (1936).

3. 'The Site of Formation of the Posterior Lobe Hormones'. E.M.K. Geiling and F.K. Oldham, *Tran. Assoc. Am. Physicians* 52, 132–136 (1937).

4. 'The Stomach Contents of Sperm Whales Caught off the West Coast of British Columbia', L.L. Robbins, Frances K. Oldham and E.M.K. Geiling, *Report of the British Columbia Provincial Museum of Natural History*, 19–21 (1937).

5. 'A Note on the Histology and Pharmacology of the Hypophysis of the Manatee (Trichechus Inumguis)'. Frances K. Oldham, D.P. McCleery and E.M.K. Geiling, *Anat. Rec.* 71, 27–32 (1938).

6. 'The Pharmacology and Anatomy of the Hypophysis of the Armadillo', Frances K. Oldham, *Anat. Rec.* 72, 265–291 (1938).

7. 'Distribution of Melanophore-Dispersing Hormone of Pituitary Gland in Anterior Lobe of Cetaceans and Armadillo'. Frances K. Oldham, Jules H. Last and E.M.K. Geiling, *Proc. Soc. Exp. Biol. and Med.,* 43, 407–410 (1940)

8. 'Appearance of the Melanophore-Expanding Hormone of Pituitary Gland in Developing Chick Embryo'. Graham Chem, Frances K. Oldham and E.M.K. Geiling, *Proc. Soc. Exp. Biol. and Med.,* 45, 310–313 (1940).

9. 'The Development of the Hypophysis of the Armadillo'. Frances K. Oldham, *Am. J. Anat.* 68, 293–315 (1941).

10. 'The Neurohypophysis', E.M.K. Geiling and Frances K. Oldham, *J. Am. Med. Assoc.* 116, 302–306 (1941).

11. 'The Melanophore Hormone', Frances K. Oldham, N.O. Calloway and E.M.K. Geiling, *Ergebnisse der Physiologis* (1941).

12. 'Cystalloids in the Hypophysis of Certain Equidae'. F.K. Oldham, *Anat. Rec.* 32, 475 (Abst.) (1942).

13. 'Studies on Antimalarial Drugs: The Distribution of Quinine in the Tissues of the Fowl'. F.E. Kelsey, Frances K. Oldham and E.M.K. Geiling, *J. Pharm. and Exper. Therap.* 78. 314–319 (1943).

14. 'Studies on Antimalarial Drugs: The Distribution of Quinine Oxidase in Animal Tissues'. F.E. Kelsey and Frances K. Oldham, Ibid., 79, 77–80 (1943).

15. 'Studies on Antimalarial Drugs: The Influence of Pregnancy on the Quinine Oxidase of Rabbit Liver'. F.K. Oldham and F.E. Kelsey, Ibid., 79, 81 (1943).

16. 'Studies on Antimalarial Drugs: The Accumulation and Excretion of Atabrine'. E.H. Dearborn, F.E. Kelsey, F.K. Oldham and E.M.K. Geiling, Ibid., 78, 120–126 (1943).

17. 'Studies on Antimalarial Drugs: The Preparations and Properties of a Metabolic Derivative of Quinine', F.E. Kelsey, E.M.K. Geiling, F.K. Oldham and E.H. Dearborn, Ibid., 80, 391–392 (1944).

18. 'Studies on Antimalarial Drugs: The Excretion of Atabrine in the Urine of the Human Subject'. F.E. Kelsey, F.K. Oldham, E.H. Dearborn, M. Silverman and E.W. Lewis, Ibid., 80, 383–385 (1944).

19. 'Studies on Antimalarial Drugs: The Effect of Malaria (Plasmodium

Gallinaceum) and of Anemia on the Distribution of Quinine in the Tissues of the Fowl'. F.K. Oldham, F.E. Kelsey, W. Cantrell and E.M.K. Geiling, Ibid., 82, 349–356 (1944).

20. 'Studies on Antimalarial Drugs: The Distribution of Atabrine in the Tissues of the Fowl and the Rabbit'. F.K. Oldham and F.E. Kelsey, Ibid., 83, 288–293 (1945).

21. 'Studies on Antimalarial Drugs: The Metabolism of Quinine and Quinidine in Birds and Mammals'. F.E. Kelsey, F.K. Oldham and E.M.K. Geiling, Ibid., 85, 170–175 (1945).

22. 'Antimalarial Activity and Toxicity of a Metabolic Derivative of Quinine'. F.E. Kelsey, F.K. Oldham, W. Cantrell and E.M.K. Geiling, *Nature* 157, 440 (1946).

23. 'Curative Effect of Plasmoquin in Plasmodium Lophuras Infections'. F.E. Kelsey, Frances K. Oldham and A.L. Gittelson, *Fed. Proc.* 5, 185 (1946).

24. *Essentials of Pharmacology*, F.K. Oldham, F.E. Kelsey and E.M.K. Geiling, J.B. Lippincott & Company, Philadelphia (1947).

25. *Essentials of Pharmacology*, 2nd Edition, F.K. Oldham, F.E. Kelsey and E.M.K. Geiling, J.B. Lippincott & Company, Philadelphia (1951).

26. *Essentials of Pharmacology*, 3rd Edition, F.K. Oldham, F.E. Kelsey and E.M.K. Geiling, J.B. Lippincott & Company, Philadelphia (1955).

27. 'Assay of Alfalfa-Containing Food Supplements for Estrogenic Activity', Cleon Schultz and Frances O. Kelsey, *Proc. S.D. Acad. Sci.*, 35, 91 (1956).

28. 'Comparative Studies on Plasma Protein Bound Iodine'. Frances O. Kelsey, Alvin Gullock and H.J. Clausen, *Proc. S.D. Acad. Sci.*, 35, 86 (1956).

29. 'Radioiodine in the Diagnosis of Thyroid Dysfunction'. Frances O. Kelsey and F. Ellis Kelsey, *S. Dak. J. Med. & Pharm.*, 9, 97 (1956).

30. 'Thyroid Activity in Hospitalized Psychiatric Patients'. Frances O. Kelsey, Alvin H. Gullock and F. Ellis Kelsey, *A.M.A. Archives of Neurology and Psychiatry*, 77, 543 (1957).

31. 'Plasma Protein-Bound Iodine in the Diagnosis of Thyroid Dysfunction'. Frances O. Kelsey and F. Ellis Kelsey, *S. Dak. J. Med. & Pharm.* 13, 275, (1960).

32. *Essentials of Pharmacology*. 4th Edition. F.K. Oldham, F.E. Kelsey and

E.M.K. Geiling, J.B. Lippincott & Company, Philadelphia (1960).

33. 'Some Observations on the Anatomy of the Beaver Pituitary'. H. J. Clausen and F. O. Kelsey, *Anat. Rec.*, 124, 274 (Abst.) (1956).

34. 'Distribution of Oxytocin, Vasopressin and Intermedin in Hypophysis of the Beaver'. F. O. Kelsey, L. Sorensen, A. A. Hagen and H. J. Clausen, *Proc. Soc. Exp. Biol. & Med.*, 95, 703 (1957).

35. 'Plasma Protein-Bound Iodine in the Beaver and Other Animals.' Frances O. Kelsey, A. Gullock and H. J. Clausen, *Acta Endocrin.*, 35, 495 (1960).

36. 'Clinical Testing of Drugs'. Frances O. Kelsey, MD, *Journal of New Drugs,* Vol. 3, No. 1, January-February 1963.

37. 'Problems Relating to Investigational Drugs'. Frances O. Kelsey, MD, *Journal of New Drugs*, Vol. 3, No. 2, March-April 1963.

38. 'The Investigational Drug Branch: A Review of Objectives and Function'. Frances O. Kelsey, MD, *Journal of New Drugs*, Vol. 3, No. 4, July-August 1963.

39. 'Symposium on Investigational Drugs'. Frances O. Kelsey, MD, *American Journal of Hospital Pharmacy*, Vol. 20, October 1963.

40. 'Drug Embryopathy – The Thalidomide Story'. Frances O. Kelsey, MD, *Maryland State Medical Journal*, December 1963.

41. 'Problems Raised for the FDA by the Occurrence of Thalidomide Embryopathy in Germany 1960–1961'. Frances O. Kelsey, MD, *South Dakota Journal of Medicine and Pharmacy*, January 1964.

42. 'Patient Consent Provisions of the Federal Food, Drug, and Cosmetic Act: Clinical Investigation in Medicine, Legal, Ethical and Moral Aspects'. Chapter 5: 336, 1963.

43. 'Control of Investigational Drugs'. Frances O. Kelsey, MD, *American Journal of Hospital Pharmacy*, Vol. 21, 320, July 1964.

44. 'Drugs in Pregnancy'. Frances O. Kelsey, MD, *Minnesota State Medical Association Journal*, Feb 1965 175–180.

45. 'IND' Review Procedure. Frances O. Kelsey, MD, presented at the 1964 Joint National Conference of the Food and Drug Administration and the Food Law Institute, Inc., *Food Drug Cosmetic Law Journal*, Vol. 20, No. 2, Feb. 1965.

46. 'First Facts About Drugs'. Frances O. Kelsey, MD, *Journal of Health-Physical Education – Recreation*, JOHPER, Vol. 36, No. 2, Feb. 1965.

47. 'Investigational Drug Branch: Intra-FDA Relationship'. Frances O. Kelsey, PhD, MD, *Food Drug Cosmetic Law Journal*, Vol. 21, No. 2, Feb. 1966, p. 102–108.

48. 'The Investigational-Drug Branch: A Look From Within', Frances O. Kelsey, MD, (Based on speech to the Food Law Institute, 9th Annual Educational Conference in D.C. 12/6/65), *Hospital Formulary Management*, March, 1966, Vol. 1, No. 2, p. 52–55.

49. 'The Evolution of New Drug Legislation'. Frances O. Kelsey, PhD, MD, Presented at the Benjamin Waterhouse History Society, Boston University School of Medicine, Boston Massachusetts, March 21, 1966, *The Boston Medical Quarterly*, September 1966.

50. 'Events Following Thalidomide'. Frances O. Kelsey, PhD, MD, Presented at the International Society of Cranio-Facial Biology, Washington, D.C. J. Dent. Res. 46: 1201–1205, 1967.

51. 'Psychopharmaka in Pregnancy'. Frances O. Kelsey, PhD, MD, Proceedings of 5th International Congress of the Collegium Internationale Neuro-Psychopharmacologicum, Washington, D.C. Mar. 1966, p. 692–696, (1967).

52. Drugs and Pregnancy. Frances O. Kelsey, PhD, MD, *Mental Retardation*, Vol. 7, No. 2, April 1969.

53. 'Drugs in Pregnancy and Their Effects on Pre- and Postnatal Development'. Frances O. Kelsey, PhD, MD, *Early Development*, Res. Publication of Association for Research in Nervous and Mental Disease, Vol. 51, Chap. 13, p. 233, 1973.

54. 'Present Guidelines for Teratogenic Studies in Experimental Animals'. Frances O. Kelsey, PhD, MD, *Congenital Defects*, New Directions in Research, 1974, Academic Press, Inc., p. 195.

55. 'Biomedical Monitoring'. Frances O. Kelsey, *The Journal of Clinical Pharmacology*, Vol. 18, No. 1, January 1978, p. 3–9.

56. 'FDA's Biomedical Research Program'. Frances O. Kelsey, *Journal of the Parenteral Drug Association*, 1979, p. 134–138.

57. 'The Importance of Epidemiology in Identifying Drugs Which May Cause Malformations – With Particular Reference to Drugs Containing Sex Hormones'. Frances O. Kelsey, *Acta Morphologica Acad. Sci. Hung.* 28 (1–2) 1980, p. 189–195.

58. 'Evaluating Clinical Investigation of Psychotropic Substances'. J.F. Wittenborn and Frances O. Kelsey, New Directions for Program Evaluation: Measuring Effectiveness, No. 11, San Francisco, Jossey-Bass, September 1981.

59. 'Regulatory Aspects of Teratology: Role of the Food and Drug Administration', Frances O. Kelsey, *Teratology* 25; 193–199, 1982.

60. 'FDA's Bioresearch Monitoring Program', Frances O. Kelsey, *Meth and Find Exptl Clin Pharmacol* 4(7), 503–508, 1982.

61. 'Volunteer Studies and Human Pharmacology-Phase I', Frances O. Kelsey, *Concepts and Strategies in New Drug Development, Clinical Pharmacology and Therapeutic Series*, Vol. 4, 123–133, 1983.

Appendix Four

TWO LETTERS TO PHYSICIANS FROM THE WM. S. MERRELL COMPANY

We give these letters unedited and verbatim, without comment. The second letter concludes with a report by Merrell about thalidomide and how Merrell sees its own role in the thalidomide disaster, with a dateline.

THE WM. S. MERRELL COMPANY
Division of Richardson-Merrell Inc. Pharmaceutical Manufacturers Since 1828 Cincinnati 15, Ohio

Frank N. Getman, President

August 10, 1962

To All Physicians:

  Last November came the first reports of a sharply rising incidence of phocomelia in some European countries and the possible association of the drug, thalidomide, with it. We at Merrell were deeply and sympathetically concerned. At that time thalidomide, under the Merrell label, was on prescription sale in Canada and undergoing clinical evaluation in the United States.

Recently this tragedy of congenital malformations has received wide publicity. Some of these reports have been confusing and some misleading. Because of this, we are outlining the facts about thalidomide and our clinical investigation of it. This report should be of interest to you and to your patients who inquire.

The facts, we believe, demonstrate:

1. Prior to the first report of congenital malformations, Merrell and its investigators had every reason to believe thalidomide was a highly useful, non-toxic substitute for the barbiturates;

2. Subsequent to such reports, Merrell has vigorously pursued a course that is in the best interests of the public welfare, both in terms of human safety and scientific and medical research.

THE WM. S. MERRELL COMPANY
Division of Richardson-Merrell Inc. Pharmaceutical Manufacturers Since 1828 Cincinnati 15, Ohio

Frank N. Getman, President

September 4, 1962

To All Physicians:

In our letter to you of August 10, 1962, we gave you the history of Merrell's connection and actions with thalidomide. As emotional reaction to early press reports begins to subside, thoughtful reanalysis is now occurring around the world.

Two examples are enclosed. One is from *The London Times* – originating in a country where thalidomide was widely used since early 1958. One illustrative of US sources – others are appearing.

Nine months have elapsed since Merrell first learned from Europe of a possible connection between thalidomide and birth defects. There have been a few reports of abnormalities in children of mothers who took thalidomide distributed under our clinical investigation program and there may be a few more. Case histories are being compiled and the facts carefully examined and appraised to determine the causative factions.

In view of the timing of our warning to active investigators last December, our own efforts to recall the drug, and the continuing effort of the FDA to assure that no supplies of thalidomide are available, we believe the critical period is now largely, if not entirely, over.

One point that has been generally overlooked to date is the therapeutic usefulness of thalidomide in certain patients. For a period exceeding three years, the English public and medical profession had extensive first-hand experience with thalidomide. It is considered so useful by British medical authorities that, although the drug was withdrawn from general distribution in England on November 28, 196, it was reinstated there on January 6, 1962 for hospital use under carefully controlled conditions.

I hope this letter may serve to bring some helpful perspective to bear upon the tragic events of the past several months.

Sincerely,
Frank N. Getman

Brief Background on Thalidomide
Thalidomide was first synthesized by Chemie Grünenthal G.m.b.H., Stolberg, West Germany, in 1953. The drug was tested in animals and then in humans. Grunenthal found it to be highly efficacious as a sedative-hypnotic, producing 'normal' sleep. The toxicity of thalidomide was extremely low in both animal and clinical testing. No LD-50 could be established.

Of particular importance, an overdose of thalidomide did not induce depression of respiration and heart action, which eliminated the possibility of accidental death and suicide through its use. Clinical reports have been published on seventeen persons who survived following ingestion of excessive amounts of the drug. One intended suicide ingested 144 times the usual dose. There are unpublished reports on many other intended suicides. No deaths from overdosage are known.

Sequence of Events
Significant events in the thalidomide history, and the facts concerning Merrell's association with the drug follow:

1953
Chemie Grünenthal synthesized thalidomide, alpha (N-phthalimide) glutarimide.

1957
Thalidomide first placed in commercial use in West Germany.

January, 1959
Merrell, under a license covering the US and Canada, commenced its own research investigation of thalidomide. At this time, thalidomide, after five years of testing and widespread use, was accepted as a safe and useful drug in Europe. It had been sold in West Germany for fifteen months without necessity for a prescription.

September 8, 1960
Merrell submitted data on animal and clinical findings to the Food and Drug Administration in the US and the Food and Drug Directorate in Canada. These findings covered more than a year and a half of testing by Merrell.

November 10, 1960 to November 30, 1961

In the United States, the Food and Drug Administration asked for additional data and details covering numerous points, such as methods of analysis for detection of the drug in the blood, added data on results in patients in the clinical studies, and these original requests and subsequent requests as rapidly as consistent with validation, point by point. This is customary under such filings. In the meantime, our clinical and animal testing was continuing. Our clinical research program concentrated on thalidomide as an hypnotic agent, where such therapy is indicated.

November 22, 1960

Merrell received notice of compliance from the Canadian Food and Drug Directorate under the new drug law.

February 14, 1961

Merrell, noting letters in *The British Medical Journal* citing instances of peripheral neuritis that were possibly toxic effects of thalidomide, wrote the English licensee for the product, Distillers Limited, asking for details.

March 6, 1961

Following exchanges of correspondence concerning the peripheral neuritis, Merrell management concluded we could not get satisfactory answers by mail and sent two Merrell scientists to Europe. They conferred with physicians in England, Scotland, and West Germany about their reports of this side effect.

March 20, 1961

We communicated to the Food and Drug Administration the information collected by our scientists in Europe.

April 1, 1961

Four months after receipt of notice of compliance from the Canadian authorities, Merrell began marketing thalidomide for prescription sale in Canada under the brand name Kevadon. Product information to physicians contained cautions concerning peripheral neuritis in the presence of long-term therapy.

[NB: Page missing.]

In terminating the clinical studies, we have collaborated closely with the Food and Drug Administration. At their request, we supplied that agency with the names of investigators in April, 1962. The FDA in turn has recently made the names of investigators in their areas available to state and local health authorities who have requested them.

While our checking and searching was in progress, we were subjected to criticism in the press for refusal to divulge the names of clinical investigators. Despite intensive pressure, Merrell maintains its firm conviction that investigators' names and patient identification were a matter of traditional medical confidence, that such facts should be divulged only to the federal government agency supervising the release of new drugs, and that the company could not in good conscience make them public.

Merrell's Further Efforts

We have pledged directly both to the Food and Drug Administration and to the American Medical Association the full cooperation and resources of Merrell in the present evaluation of thalidomide's potential teratogenicity and in the search both for other causal factors and, if possible, for preventive measures. In the past month we have made available to the FDA the case record material which was available to us from Europe.

We will, of course, cooperate fully in the program of the newly established Commission on Drug Safety created by the Pharmaceutical Manufacturers Association and headed by Dr Lowell T. Coggeshall to develop new guidelines for research and testing on the basis of the most advanced scientific knowledge.

At the same time we have expanded our own laboratory research program into the teratogenic effects of various agents. Much remains to be learned in this area, most specifically in regard to thalidomide itself.

We have not at any time minimized the possible relationship between thalidomide and congenital malformations. We hope this series of events will lead to better scientific understanding of the development of the human embryo and to progress in preventing fetal abnormalities whatever the cause.

We plan to do everything in our power to help assure this outcome.

An Appraisal of Merrell's Efforts

On August 1st, a Senate subcommittee studying broad problems of medical communication held a hearing at which much attention was devoted to thalidomide. George P. Larrick, commissioner of the Food and Drug Administration, and Dr Frances O. Kelsey, the FDA medical officer who handled the new drug application, both appeared before the subcommittee.

Following the hearing, Senator Hubert Humphrey, chairman of the subcommittee, told the Associated Press that Merrell had acted responsibly throughout and 'complied with every regulation'.

I hope this report has been of interest to you.

Sincerely,
Frank N. Getman

ACKNOWLEDGEMENTS

We would like to thank the following people for their help with our work on this book:

Our primary thanks are to Dr John Swann of the FDA, who knew Frances personally and whose help, from the start of this project, has been absolutely vital.

We also thank most sincerely Sir Harold Evans for agreeing to write the Preface. The movie *Attacking the Devil* (2014), about Sir Harold's campaign to win compensation for British thalidomide victims, is absolutely riveting and has been made available on streaming services.

Our sincere gratitude to Margaret Dowley, MBE, for her hard work transcribing the Dictaphone tapes and her help with document copy-typing, and also to Helen Komatsu for the excellent secretarial help she provided at short notice.

The very beginning of the book, about how society sees poets, was suggested by a passage in the memoirs of Kingsley Amis about his recollections of the very start of a lecture given by Lord David Cecil.

At the James Madison Memorial Building of the Library of Congress in Washington, D.C., James was given great and unstinting help by Melinda Friend. Many thanks also to Frederick J. Augustyn, J. Richard Crout, Will Newkirk, and Jeffrey Flannery, Joseph Jackson, Patrick Kerwin, Bruce Kirby, Melissa Lindberg, Edith Sandler, and Lewis Wyman of the Library of Congress, and to Briony Kapoor, James Walker, Rupert Essinger, to the general manager and staff of the Fairfax at Embassy Row Hotel, Washington, D.C., and Lu Mistry and her colleagues at the Regency Hotel in Leicester, England, where some of this book was written.

Our additional warm thanks to all of the following: Ruth Blue of the Thalidomide Society; Laura Colombi; Robyn Drury; the late Agnes Donnellon; Angela Donnellon; Daisy Donnellon and Kev Donnellon; Mark Edmondson; Francesca Garratt, who helped to inspire the research and writing of this book; Dr Laurence Green; Andrew Greet; Professor Charles Lewis; and Mandy Masters. Our great gratitude to Matthew Kelly and Chantelle Sturt at Wellspring in the US, and to Chrissy McMorris, Fenton Coulthurst, Jessicca Gofton and Jezz Palmer at The History Press.

J.E. & S.K.

INDEX

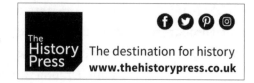